THE NEW DEFINITIVE
GRAIN-FREE BAKING BOOK

From the beginning, Sweet Laurel has been about making sweet things simple. The recipes here are indulgent yet healthful. They use just a few quality ingredients to create delicious desserts that benefit your body; all of them are paleo, and many are vegan and raw. From **MATCHA SANDWICH COOKIES** to **SALTED LEMON MERINGUE PIE** to classic **GERMAN CHOCOLATE CAKE**, these treats are at once uncomplicated, beautiful, and satisfying, made only with wholesome ingredients such as almonds, coconut, cacao, and dates. Here, too, are basic staple recipes, like grain-free vanilla extract and vegan caramel, and fancy finishes, like paleo sprinkles and dairy-free ice cream.

Whether you're looking for simpler recipes, seeking a better approach to dessert, or struggling with an allergy that has prevented you from enjoying sweets, *Sweet Laurel* will change the way you bake.

SWEET LAUREL

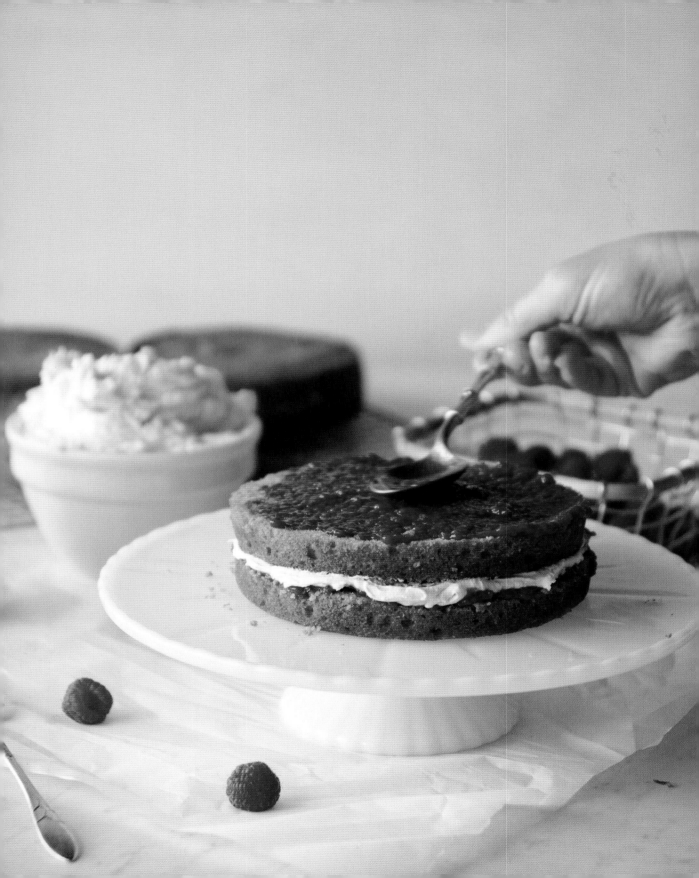

SWEET LAUREL

RECIPES FOR
WHOLE FOOD, GRAIN-FREE DESSERTS

LAUREL GALLUCCI AND CLAIRE THOMAS

FOREWORD BY LAUREN CONRAD

PHOTOGRAPHY BY CLAIRE THOMAS

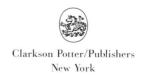

Clarkson Potter/Publishers
New York

TO OUR DARLING SONS, NICO AND JAMES

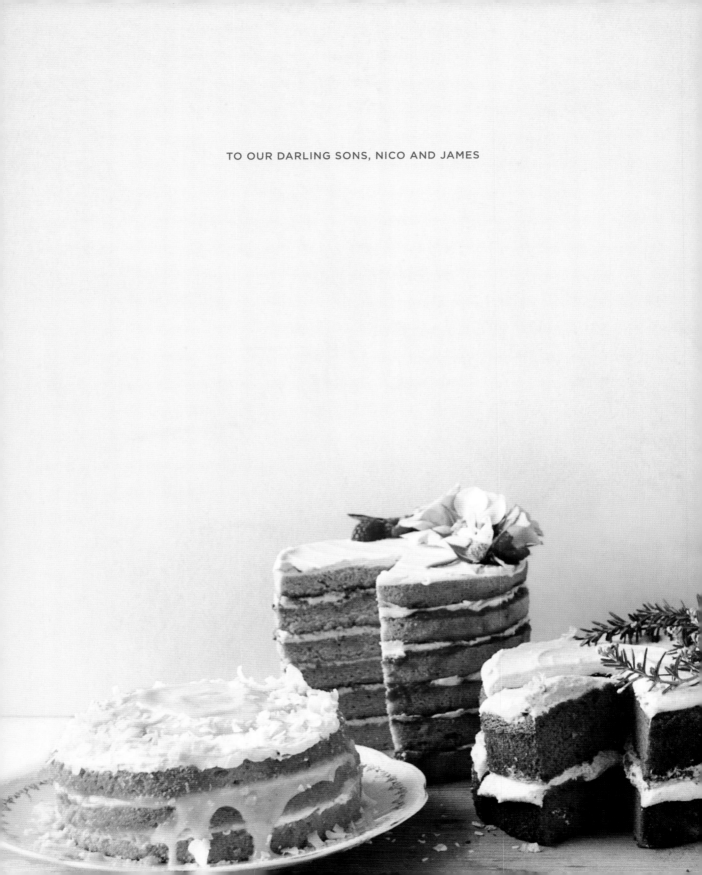

CONTENTS

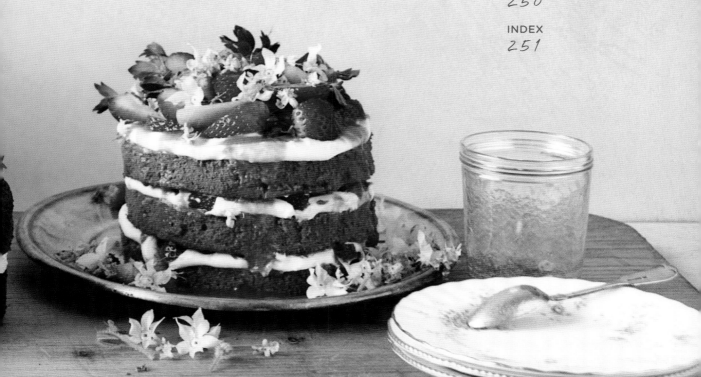

I love cake. There, I said it.

And pie, too. OK, top anything with whipped cream and I'm in. Honestly, I can't remember the last meal I had where I didn't "save room for dessert." Who knew that years later my family and my own diet would have to change completely. But don't worry, we all get that slice of cake in the end.

You can imagine my predicament when on our second date, my now-husband dropped a real bombshell. No, he wasn't married or a felon. It was worse. He said he wasn't "a dessert person."

Excuse me? Recognizing my shock, he offered one exception: chocolate chip cookies. Come on, that's not real . . . Everyone likes chocolate chip cookies!

I know what you're thinking: I still had time to get out.

Unfortunately, he's handsome, smart, and we share the same lame sense of humor. He also has great hair . . . Seriously, it's like Disney prince hair. I decided to stick it out, but had to reverse this terrible transgression—which I did! In fact, he credits me with his sweet tooth. However, our happily-ever-after was short-lived, because William suffered from sinus issues that could only be reversed by cutting dairy from his diet . . . entirely.

Do you know which foods contain dairy? Basically *everything*—especially desserts.

My next step was to begin living a double life. I feigned sympathy while whispering dessert orders, I snuck into the kitchen to eat ice cream sandwiches over the sink, I pretended it was lemonade in my cup and not a milkshake. I mean, I needed to keep living my life!

But during my pregnancy everything changed. William's feelings about desserts (or otherwise) became of little consequence, because only one thing could cure my constant nausea: sweets. I no longer had the energy to hide our forbidden love, and it didn't take me long to start binge-eating ice cream straight from the carton . . . on our couch. And once our son arrived things got even crazier. Did you know breastfeeding burns 500 calories a day? Cupcakes for everyone! (I mean, except William.)

Since all scandalous affairs have disastrous ends, something awful happened. Our son started having tummy problems; it appeared he was . . . lactose intolerant. In order to continue breastfeeding, I'd need to cut out all dairy. I wanted to keep Liam breastfeeding a little longer, so I had to adjust my diet.

You know what they say about payback, right? I watched everyone around me, night after night, indulge in dessert. It was merciless.

Enter, Claire and Laurel. I have enjoyed Sweet Laurel's delicious concoctions over the years and not only do they make some of the best-tasting sweets, they also make some of the most beautiful. I can't overstate this: they make stunning desserts. Apparently, they're also healthier too, but I never even got to that part . . . Frosting and a garden rose? Yeah, I'm in.

I was only a few weeks into my dairy-free gloom when Claire asked if I would write this foreword. When she sent me the book, I nearly jumped out of my chair when I saw those two little words: DAIRY-FREE. Did this book really have the potential to give my dairy-free saga a happy ending? Could it rescue us from these lacto-free shackles?

I started small: coconut whipped cream. I followed the recipe carefully, and it fluffed up in the bowl like a cloud: pillowy and white, a little piece of heaven. I knew it would look lovely, but how would it taste?

Wonderful! Frothy, light, and delightfully creamy—but there wasn't any cream! My future sweet life suddenly didn't seem so bleak. But I needed to know this wasn't just a fluke; I had to test something else. I set my sights on the poppy seed cake.

Now, my mother-in-law's poppy seed cake is legendary and no one dares challenge it. I had to choose between family and dessert, and I don't know if I can actually admit that it was . . . better. It was better. *Sweet Laurel*'s recipe was better. (To my mother-in-law, I love you and please remember I gave you a grandchild.)

Feeling a natural-sugar-induced, dessert-filled high, I decided to embark on the truest of tests: chocolate chip cookies. My husband arrived home just as they came out of the oven, filling the air with the sort of warm, chocolatey goodness that could definitely convince him to handle the midnight feeding. The entire first batch of gooey perfection disappeared before the next sheet was even in the oven. I knew then that we had witnessed a miracle; we had been saved! Thank you, Claire and Laurel!

While this book is an incredible resource for those looking to omit grains, dairy, and refined sugar from their diets, it's also filled with simple-to-execute recipes for beautiful food everyone can enjoy without feeling like they're sacrificing. Not to mention, creating sweets that are tasty *and* nourishing might just give us all one more excuse to "save room for dessert."

LAUREN CONRAD

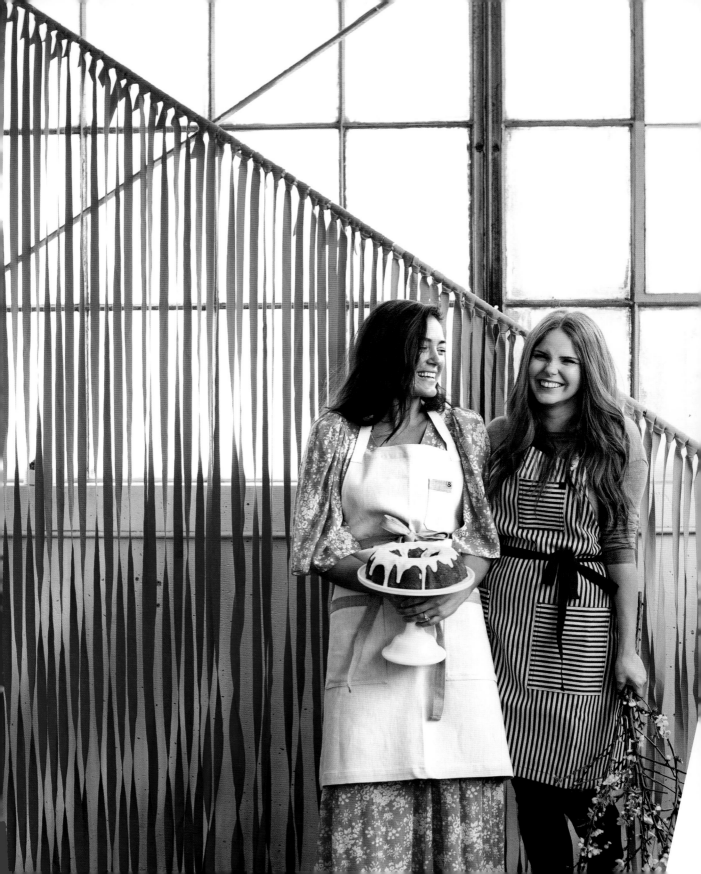

INTRODUCTION

Sweet Laurel is a story of friendship and passion, told not through words, but through cake. It's our story.

Let's back up. Baking has always created memories for us. Laurel's love of baking started when she was four or five years old. She made banana bread with her mom, and tasting the batter, was instantly hooked. Her nanny let her help make homemade snacks, and with her grandfather she made stacks of pancakes that were so tall, she couldn't see over them. Baking became her hobby, and soon she was old enough to gain freedom in the kitchen.

Ten years later, Laurel had shelves of cookbooks and stacks of culinary magazines, the covers threadbare from flipping pages thousands of times. But her love for baking came to a dramatic halt when her life was rocked by the derailing diagnosis of an autoimmune condition, Hashimoto's disease, and a digestive disorder. The doctor told her she would never eat chocolate cake again. But Laurel's desire to bake remained, so she refused to accept that answer. How could she enjoy the life ahead without grains, especially gluten, dairy, and refined sugar? After all, nearly all Laurel's homemade recipes contained at least one of these now-forbidden ingredients.

Laurel's distress did not last long. Soon she learned the beauty of whole food ingredients: almonds, coconut, cacao, organic eggs, dates . . . and many more she never imagined could play a role in baking. She began making treats with the foods that nourished her, keeping the recipes simple. Laurel found that when working with nutrient-dense foods, fillers, thickeners, and other undesirable additions were not necessary. With just seven to ten staple ingredients, Laurel created recipes that brought back memories of her childhood baking, but they were so much more nourishing.

A few months later, Laurel shared a grain-free, refined-sugar-free, dairy-free chocolate caramel cake with her friend Claire. Laurel was an educator and home baker and Claire was a food blogger, so we had connected over a love of emotional baking. Claire has no food allergies or sensitivities, so when Laurel offered her the slice of cake, she didn't provide any context. While Claire was licking her fork, Laurel smiled and asked, "So, you liked it?"

Then Laurel dropped the bomb. This delicious chocolate caramel cake with fudge frosting was completely devoid of what Claire thought were her favorite ingredients. It was wholesome, nutritious, and autoimmune friendly. Claire was floored—she had been constantly disappointed by gluten-free or vegan baked options, and was a self-described carb snob. The textures and flavors always seemed a bit off, like a photocopy of a photocopy of the thing they claimed to be. That was the moment when we knew we had to do more with that chocolate cake.

With our mouths full and plates clean, we decided to start a bakery together: Sweet Laurel.

The next few months were spent baking, tasting, and then baking some more. Inspired by the simple recipes Laurel had developed, Claire began decorating the cakes with small bouquets of edible flowers. Anything too fussy or polished just didn't feel right. Our naked cakes, with luscious frosting, fresh jam, or gooey caramel dripping down the sides, were topped with a few organic roses, blossoming herbs, or whatever we could find at the farmer's market. The Sweet Laurel Look—simple, feminine, and a bit romantic—was set.

But at that point we were still just two girlfriends and a bunch of cakes. We discovered what would set Sweet Laurel apart at a lunch hosted by designer and tastemaker Jenni Kayne. We weren't just going to drop off some cakes for the ladies to enjoy; we were going to teach a class as well. Claire had done some demos at Jenni's before and Laurel's previous career was as a teacher, so we figured this experiment would be fun. We were an intimate eight sitting on kitchen stools around Jenni's counter, making it more like hanging out with girlfriends than a typical class. As the class went on, we were peppered with questions: What's the benefit of using coconut oil? Is grain-free the same as gluten-free? Why doesn't everything taste like maple syrup if we're using it in everything? Laurel answered all the questions with ease. The women marveled at our simple two-step method for baking the cake, and passed slices around to taste. Leftovers were promptly wrapped up for them to share with their children at home.

As we were cleaning up, one of the guests stopped by on her way out. "Do you guys do private classes?" We glanced at each other and in unison replied, "Yes!" We hadn't really discussed it, but as people asked us about sharing recipes, catering children's birthday parties, and hosting private classes, we realized something important was going on. We weren't opening a bakery for anonymous customers to grab a slice of cake; we were providing a service. You know what they say: "Give a girl a cake and she'll eat for one day. Teach a girl to bake and . . ."

We discovered that education and empowerment were becoming the cornerstones of our business. Without them, Sweet Laurel would just be another bakery—one that happens to be grain-free. It's our constant interaction and relationships with customers, their needs, and their questions that define who we are as a company. This cookbook is a continuation of that dynamic. For everyone who can't make it to a workshop or a private class, we have collected our recipes and knowledge in this book. Our secrets, our tips, our experiences—they're all here.

From the beginning, Sweet Laurel has been about making sweet things simple. We aim to take the drama and judgment out of the healthy living experience by providing our customers with beautiful, delicious, and satisfying desserts; our followers with easy recipes and tips; and our community with workshops and classes. Our goal is to create an empowering, transformative, and sweet experience that makes you excited to take your next bite. Our food is indulgent yet healthful. It's about loving the food you eat instead of punishing yourself for craving it.

Our book will give you an outlet to enjoy great-tasting grain-free, gluten-free, refined-sugar-free, dairy-free, gum-free, soy-free, and filler-free recipes that benefit your body. All of our treats are paleo, and some are vegan, raw, or nut-free as well. We've marked those that are vegan and nut-free with symbols at the tops of the recipes: V and NF. Most of the recipes revolve around five core ingredients, and none of them are the wacky additives you find in most "healthy" desserts. Whether you're looking for a simpler way to bake, a better approach to dessert, or a solution to an allergy that has prevented you from enjoying sweets, we want to change the way you bake.

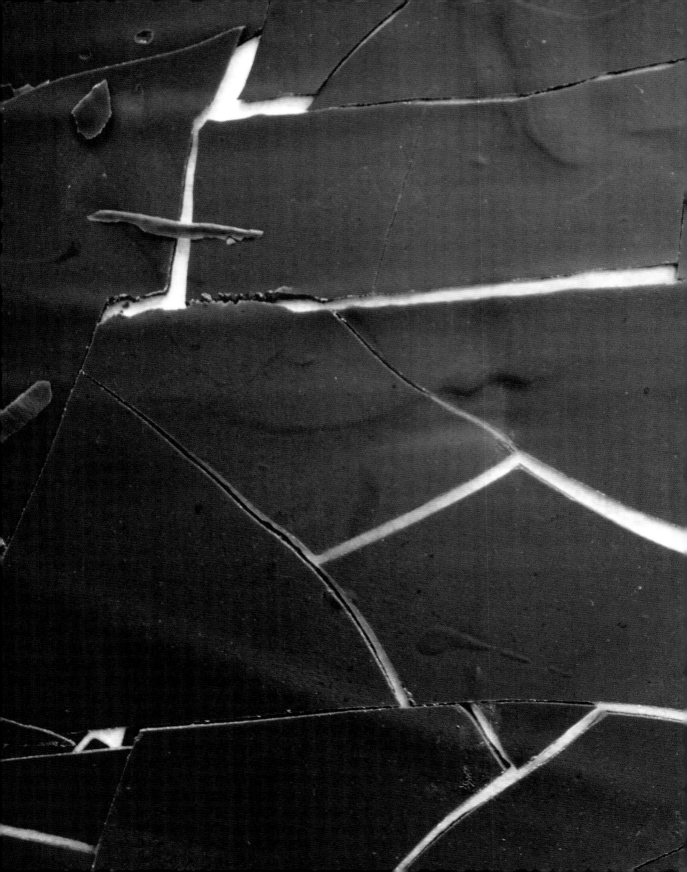

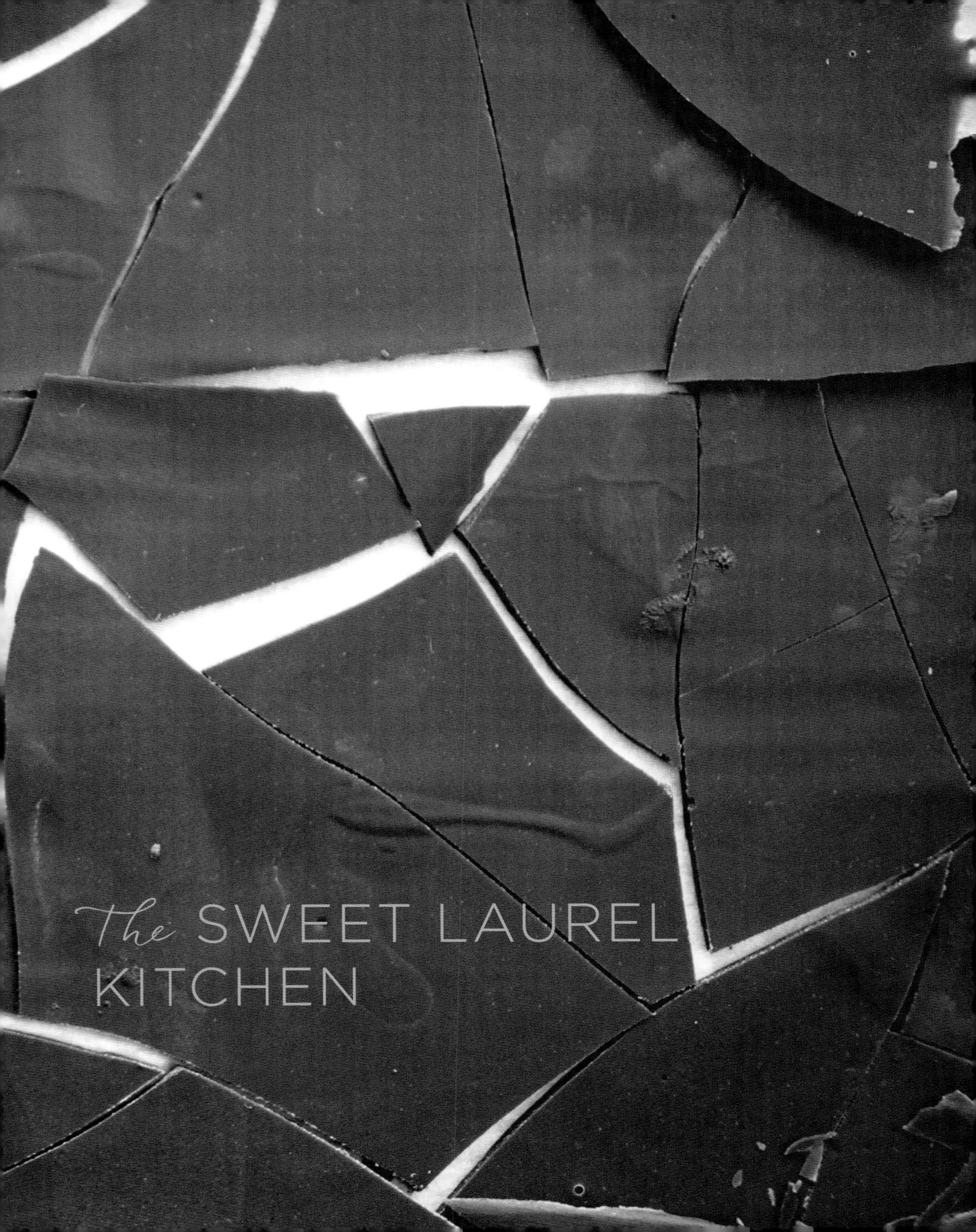
The SWEET LAUREL
KITCHEN

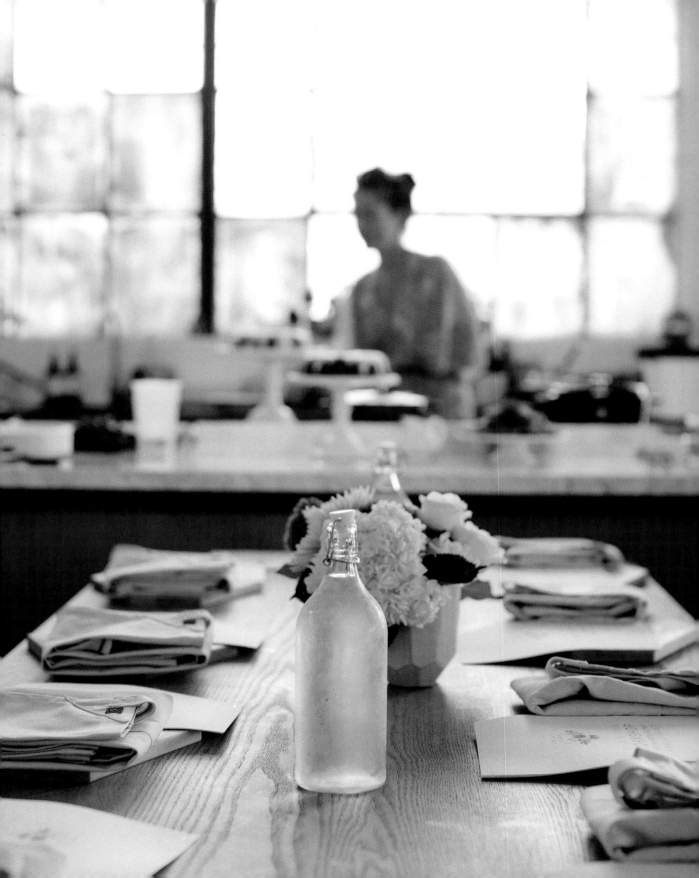

THE SWEET LAUREL METHOD

At Sweet Laurel, we work with nutrient-dense, organic ingredients. We don't take shortcuts because our recipes are so simple that we don't need to. Working with whole food ingredients is not only beneficial to your body, but is also one of the keys to making delicious baked goods. Our secret to moist, light, and perfectly delicious grain-free desserts lies in our five principles.

1. KEEP IT SIMPLE. That means no more than five core ingredients in any given recipe. You can stock your kitchen with almond flour, coconut oil, organic eggs, maple syrup, and Himalayan pink salt and make practically any recipe in this book. (See page 16 for more specific information.) Gluten-free and dairy-free baking is often overcomplicated, sometimes involving several different flours and added gums or fillers. Not here! "Could it be simpler?" is the question we always ask ourselves. You'll see a lot of familiar ideas in our approach, just made simpler.

2. KEEP IT WHOLE. Use ingredients that are as close to their natural form, or as whole as possible, with nothing added. Almond flour, for example, is simply made from grinding blanched almonds. Maple syrup is made by boiling down the sap of maple trees. We love Himalayan pink salt because it doesn't have bleach or anticaking agents. Processed foods often have trace ingredients that can not only change the outcome of your recipe, but also trigger a sensitivity (gluten, for instance, pops up in tons of processed foods because it binds ingredients together). We believe eating the foods that nature offers us is important—they are far better for your body, plus you have better control in the kitchen because you know exactly what you're working with.

3. KEEP IT BALANCED. Baking is chemistry. When you remove grains, sugar, and dairy, you have to replace those ingredients with ones that have similar behaviors. Once you get the hang of it, you can tackle any sweet treat. Our recipes have been developed and tested over years of research and they do not play by the typical baking rules. The Sweet Laurel Method has its own set of rules, yes, but they are far more user friendly. By following the recipes in this book, you will see how our ingredients balance out one another to yield successful results.

4. KEEP IT STRESS-FREE. Our low-tech, as in low technique, approach sets us apart from classic bakeries. If you have a bowl and a whisk, you can create almost every single one of our recipes. We have long used baking as a stress reliever—it's fun and meditative. Our less complicated, simplicity-forward style of baking encourages a relaxing kitchen environment.

5. KEEP IT BEAUTIFUL. Our sweets are well known for their romantic aesthetic. Our baked goods are not just filled with beautiful ingredients—they are also designed to show off those ingredients. In "The Grand Finale" on page 233, we'll share our method for taking a simple cake and turning it into an eye-catching dessert. We don't use chemical-based food colorings or sugar-filled decor; we use nature: food-based colorings (see page 210), organic florals, and fruit. It is truly beauty from the inside out. All of our decorating techniques can be done with no experience or skill in decorating, so don't worry if you've never handled a pastry bag before.

WHAT'S INSIDE

We believe in using the highest quality, nutrient-dense ingredients to create the most delicious and flavorful baked goods. Traditionally, a baker's pantry uses flour, white sugar, and butter to create the base for most desserts. But when a doctor's orders delete all three of those mainstays from one's diet, alternatives are required. Our grain-free, refined-sugar-free, and dairy-free pantry is based on an anti-inflammatory and holistic approach to health.

WHAT'S THE DIFFERENCE BETWEEN GRAIN-FREE AND GLUTEN-FREE?

This is a bit like asking, What's the difference between a square and a rectangle? Gluten is a protein found in some grains (wheat, rye, and oats, for instance), so since Sweet Laurel is grain-free, it means we're gluten-free, too.

But why remove gluten or grains to begin with? Gluten is a protein that adds structure to breads and baked goods, and can also be found in processed foods to help bind ingredients, like in canned soups and sauces. For many people, this protein is inflammatory, adding to digestive and autoimmune issues. Gluten-free recipes can rely on other grains, like rice and corn, but at Sweet Laurel we go a step further, removing all grains from our recipes. A grain-free diet has been known to help with digestive disorders and autoimmune diseases, as in Laurel's case.

Quinoa, amaranth, and buckwheat technically are not grains, however, we do not include them in our recipes, but instead rely on nut and coconut flours.

OUR CORE INGREDIENTS

Almond Flour
Almond flour is nutritionally dense, typically made from almonds that have been blanched (brown peel removed). Compared with other tree nuts, almonds are higher in fiber, calcium, vitamin E, riboflavin, and niacin, not to mention offering a solid amount of protein and other nutrients like magnesium (one ounce of almonds provides 6 grams of protein and 4 grams of fiber); plus, like other nuts, they are low-glycemic (how your body reacts to sugar; high-glycemic food means a sugar spike and crash). But just because almonds and other nuts are packed with nutrients doesn't mean they're a low-calorie food. Most nuts contain a fairly high amount of fat, with about 14 grams per one-ounce serving, but about two-thirds of that is heart-healthy, monounsaturated fat. The combination of fat, fiber, and protein is why almond flour is such a fabulous foundation for our cakes. It has some structure from the protein, is always moist from the fat, and has the added nutritional benefit of all those vitamins, minerals, and fiber. This is why every slice of a Sweet Laurel cake is so filling and satisfying. The calories are sweet but they're certainly not empty. Almond flour is easy to find in any grocery store, but we share our own recipe on page 37. If you are allergic to almonds, you can substitute hazelnut flour or cashew flour in our recipes. If you're allergic to nuts, you can substitute coconut flour, with some additional adjustments (see page 19).

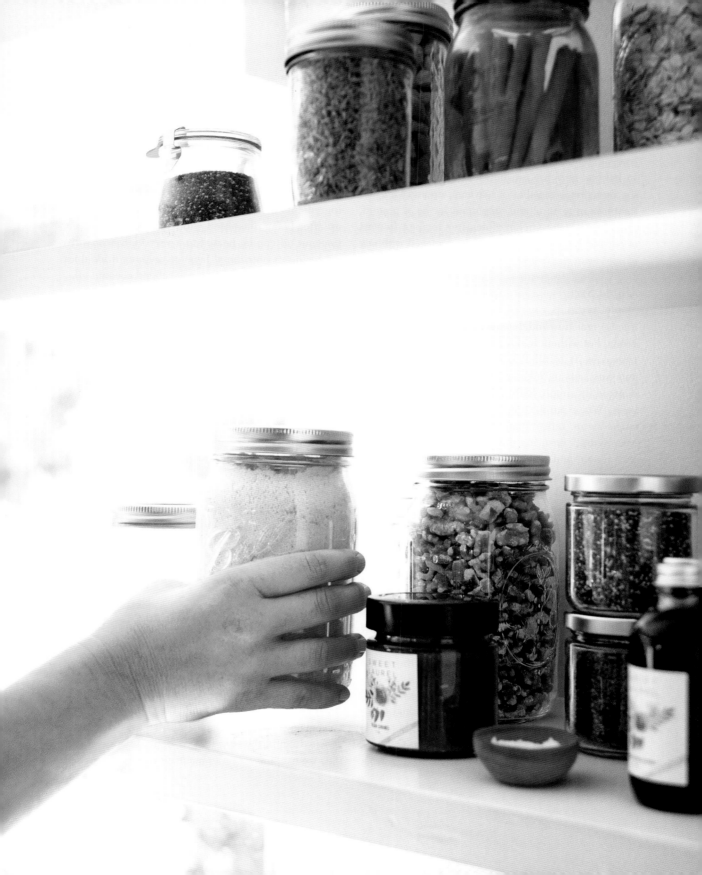

soak them in hot water for about 30 minutes or until they're tender. Drain and pat them dry before using.

Honey

Honey is a great alternative sweetener and can be used instead of maple syrup in any of our recipes. However, we tend to use less of it because heating honey will diminish its nutritional benefits. Raw, lightly filtered honey contains pollen, twenty-two amino acids, twenty-seven minerals, and plenty of vitamins. Despite tasting super sweet, it registers lower on the glycemic index than sugar. We'll use raw honey in recipes that don't require heating, but if we do use honey in a baking recipe, we'll sometimes finish it with additional raw honey. It adds a lovely final punch of sweet and some of those extra benefits, too. Raw honey can crystallize, but this doesn't mean it has gone bad. We like to spread thick, crystallized honey on toast—it's delicious!

Cacao (100% Unsweetened Cacao Powder and 100% Cacao Unsweetened Baking Chocolate)

Our recipes call for both cacao powder and whole unsweetened cacao, in bar form, for baking. Chocolate is made from cacao, but for our recipes, we use only unsweetened, 100 percent cacao. This means that a typical bar of dark chocolate is not a good substitute for our recipes, as we work with cacao in its pure form. Chocolate, even bittersweet chocolate, contains additives such as sugar, milk, and binders like soy lecithin. If you have trouble finding pure cacao, just look at the ingredient list on the back—100 percent cacao will not list any other ingredients. Bars labeled as unsweetened chocolate or baking chocolate often are 100 percent cacao, so simply double-check before purchasing. Cacao is renowned for its energy-boosting abilities. If you've ever had a few nibbles of 100 percent cacao, you already know about this energy boost! Laurel eats it every day while her husband sips on his morning cup of coffee.

Gelatin

Gelatin is used in many of our custard pies and also our delicious Marshmallows (page 28). We like to use grass-fed beef gelatin, sometimes referred to as "collagen," as it's high in protein. You can also find soy-based alternatives; we don't use them in our baking because Laurel is soy sensitive, but they will work fine. Great Lakes is our favorite brand.

Baking Powder

We make our own baking powder (see page 33) because the store-bought stuff typically contains cornstarch and aluminum, and honestly, it's super easy to mix up a batch.

Baking Soda

Like baking powder, baking soda is a leavening agent, but much more powerful. It also counteracts acidic ingredients used in baking. We use natural baking soda, meaning baking soda that has been mined rather than lab created, such as the Bob's Red Mill brand, in our recipes.

Lemon Juice

You can of course buy lemon juice at the store, but it's super easy to make—just squeeze lemons into a bowl while straining out the pulp and seeds. Whenever we call for it, we mean the fresh stuff.

Apple Cider Vinegar

Apple cider vinegar is fermented apple juice, and we like to use it in recipes needing extra brightness. Our delicious Savory Turmeric Bread (page 70), for example, gets a lovely bite from the added acid. Fermented ingredients were a huge part of Laurel's gut health recovery after her diagnosis, and apple cider vinegar is a delicious and easy way to add some beneficial bacteria and enzymes to your diet. The acetic acid in apple cider vinegar has the ability to kill dangerous "bad" bacteria and at the same time foster the growth of beneficial "good" bacteria. Look for raw, "cold-pressed" brands that have sediment in the bottom, like Bragg's.

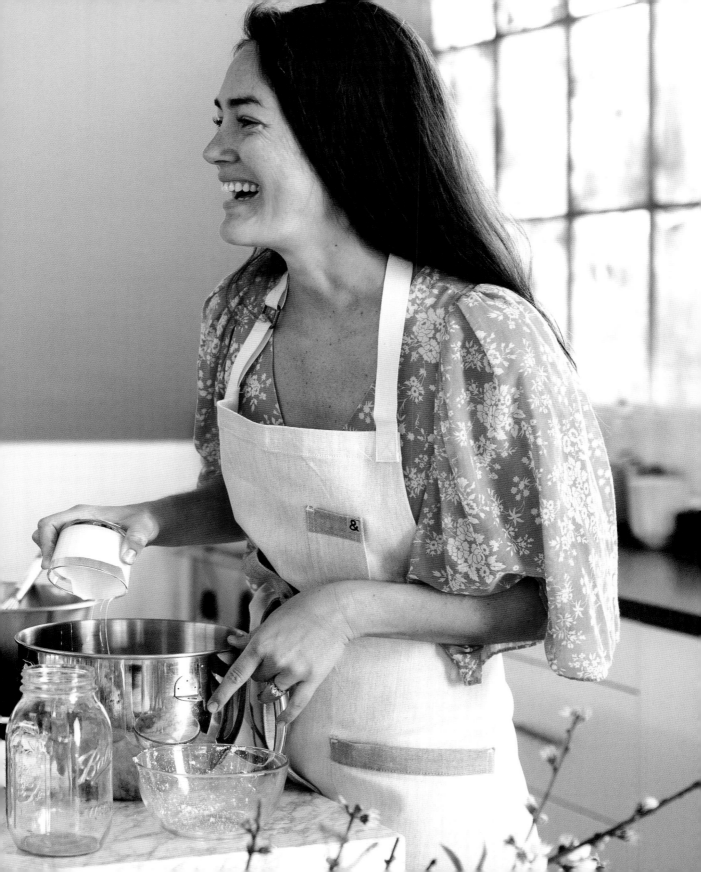

Grass-Fed Ghee

We don't use ghee often in our recipes, but for getting cake to slip out of a Bundt pan, you can't find anything better. Ghee is made by melting butter and then removing all of the milk solids, rendering it lactose- and casein-free. Choosing grass-fed over conventional ghee is an easy choice for us, as grass-fed ghee contains vitamin K (good for heart health) and 25 percent medium- and short-chain fatty acids (like the fat found in coconut milk), which your body metabolizes more easily and faster than butter. It can also be used to replace coconut oil if you tolerate dairy well, as the milk solids that contain lactose have been removed.

Vanilla Extract

At Sweet Laurel we make our own vanilla extract to ensure it's not only gluten- and grain-free, but also full of flavor. Store-bought vanilla extracts often include unnecessary fillers and grain- and gluten-containing alcohols. We make ours with tequila (a grain-free alcohol) and freshly sliced vanilla beans and seeds. Our version (see page 33) not only adds delicious flavor, but also guarantees a gluten-free baked good!

Spices

Cinnamon is our favorite anti-inflammatory spice to add to treats, so you will see it a lot in this cookbook. It can lower your body's blood sugar levels—and tastes great. Our other favorite spices are turmeric, cayenne, and ginger. Not only do they give our recipes a kick, but they also provide digestive and anti-inflammatory benefits. We recommend keeping all of these on hand.

Nuts and Nut Butters

It didn't take long for Laurel to discover that nuts and nut butters are powerful stand-ins for grains. Nuts are loaded with good fats and protein, and compared with grains, contain far fewer carbohydrates. Our first choice in most recipes is almond butter; however, hazelnut and cashew butters work beautifully, too. These are widely available, but easy to make yourself (see page 38). If you're allergic to nuts, sunflower seed butter is a wonderful option.

Our homemade versions of nut butters and nut milk can be found in "Our Essential Recipes." Two caveats: First, always choose fresh, raw nuts. This helps the butter last longer, but it also keeps the flavor light and clean. And second, yes, you really do have to soak the nuts first even though it's an extra step. Not only does it make the nut puree creamier, but it also greatly reduces the phytic acid (also found in grains and legumes), which can inhibit your body's absorption of minerals and enzymes.

Matcha

Matcha is a powdered green tea that is predominantly grown and produced in Japan. The green tea leaves are shaded from the sun for the last few weeks of their growth, increasing the chlorophyll content and creating a deep and vibrant green color. Then the leaves are carefully ground into a fine, antioxidant-rich powder—sixty times more powerful than spinach. If you've tasted matcha before, it's probably been as a frothy cup of hot tea or in ice cream. Matcha is very potent, so a little goes a long way. We adore the flavor in our desserts and the rich color in our frostings. Be sure to use the freshest you can find and store it in a cool, dry place. Otherwise, the powder can turn a bit yellow and sad, rather than bright green.

Fruit

Organic berries, apples, pineapple, cherries, lemons, and many more delectable types of fruit are sprinkled throughout our recipes. We love highlighting fruits in our baked goods, allowing them to fully express themselves without hiding their unique flavors behind too much added sweetener or other ingredients. If finding high-quality fresh fruit is challenging, check your grocer's freezer—many of our recipes work perfectly well with frozen fruit. Just be sure it's organic and from a good source.

OUR ESSENTIAL TOOLS

You don't need much equipment to make these beautiful recipes. Here's what we recommend having on hand. They're not all essential, but they will make your life a little easier.

A Bowl and a Whisk

In truth, almost every recipe in this book can be made with a bowl and a whisk. We recommend a very large bowl to be sure you have plenty of room to work. We tend to use a Pyrex glass bowl set or plain stainless steel bowls. When you cut out the gluten you lose structure but you end up with a batter that is impossible to overbeat. As long as the batter or dough is fully blended, you're good to go!

A Really Good Blender

There are a lot of fabulous blenders out there and at a lot of different price points. This can definitely be a big-ticket item, but a good blender can be a lifesaver in the kitchen. Making almond milk takes half the time it usually does, and almond butter turns out creamy instead of gritty. Also, a good blender will make separated coconut milk smooth immediately. Vitamix and KitchenAid are our favorite brands. A lower-price-point blender may mean you need to take more time, or sieve ingredients between blendings.

Rubber Spatula

Other than being necessary for mixing, folding, and pouring, spatulas are key for scraping the bottom of the bowl—we hate waste! We like tiny rubber spatulas for scraping between the blades of a blender. Trust us, using a regular-sized spatula to clean out a blender is a nightmare.

Offset Spatula

Our favorite tool for getting those perfectly imperfect zaftig curves in our frosting is the offset spatula. It looks like a flat butter knife with a little bend up to the handle. No frosting on your fingers and more pressure control.

Food Processor

Similar to a really good blender, a food processor is ideal for quick chopping and perfect blending of thicker ingredients, like our Vegan Caramel (page 40).

Parchment Paper

Whether you're lining a baking sheet of cookies, rolling up a block of date paste, or separating layers of just-baked cake, humble parchment paper is a kitchen necessity. Plus, it's one of the few things almond flour *doesn't* stick to!

Silicone Mats and Cake Molds

Silicone mats and molds are immensely useful. Since we don't use wheat flour to coat problematic pans, we usually turn to silicone to help with cakes that don't want to budge (though parchment and liberal amounts of coconut oil are good choices, too). You can also use silicone mats to line your baking sheets.

Pastry Blender

For making quick breads and piecrusts, you can't beat a pastry blender. Using your warm fingertips to mix the ingredients can cause the fat to melt, making your pastry heavy. But with a pastry blender, you can combine everything while keeping the dough very cold, leading to a more tender, lighter result.

Nylon Nut-Milk Bag

We don't usually go for single-use tools, but this one is too good and cheap not to have in our kitchen drawer. Reusable, strong, and efficient, a milk bag makes straining nut milk much easier than with cheesecloth, and you can throw it in the washer. It's perfect for our recipe on page 37.

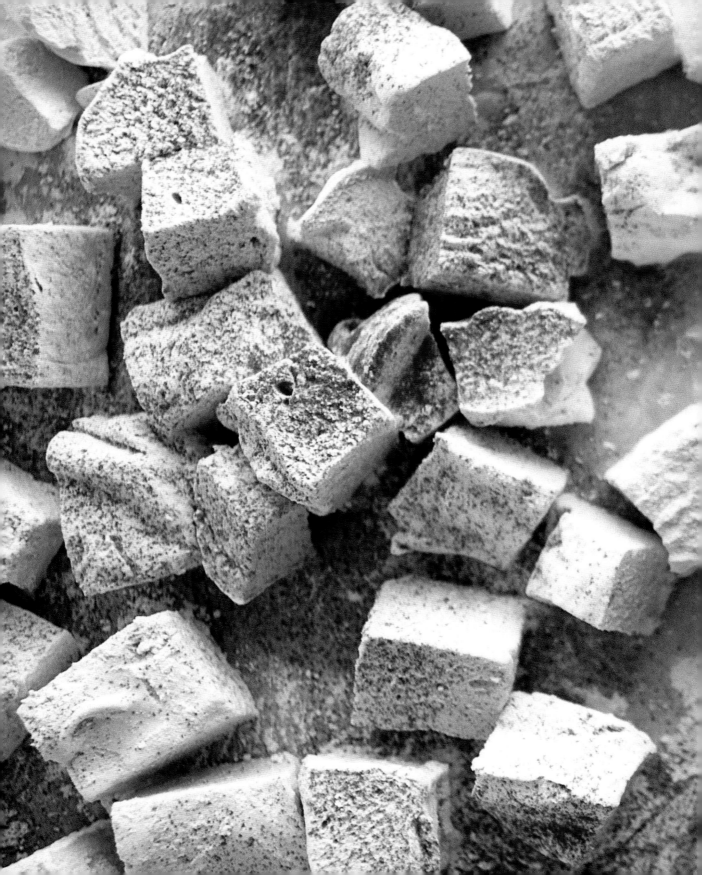

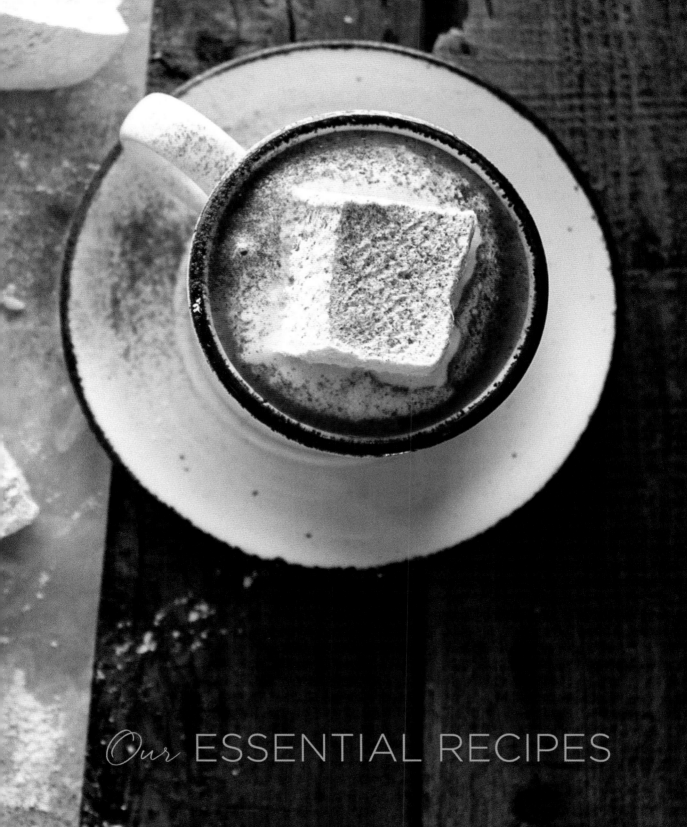

Our ESSENTIAL RECIPES

The foundational recipes in this chapter are the bedrock of the Sweet Laurel approach to baking. Without them, you won't be able to make many of the recipes in the book. Some of these ingredients can be purchased at the market (coconut yogurt, vegan chocolate chips, etc.), but we recommend making them yourself at least once so you can see the difference in taste and quality. Particularly if you have food allergies, being able to completely control what's in your food is paramount, and store-bought equivalents for our recipes in this section—such as grain-free vanilla extract—are hard to find in the market.

This chapter is where we reveal the secrets to our baked goods. When you remove butter (for moisture and tenderness), sugar (for stability, caramelization, and crunch), and flour (for structure), the right texture can seem elusive to even the most experienced home baker. Without these three ingredients, cake can become heavy, piecrust chewy, custard rubbery, and bread crumbly.

So how is Sweet Laurel different? Well, as we discuss on page 15, we don't use any weird stuff. Most of the ingredients we call for will be familiar to any home cook, and we always try to use them in their whole, simple form. This usually leads to simpler recipes, too. We meet the challenges that arise from replacing conventional ingredients or techniques with our grain-free, refined-sugar-free, and dairy-free alternatives by finding new ways to balance moisture, texture, lightness, and stability. In our style of baking, the simplest solution is usually the best one.

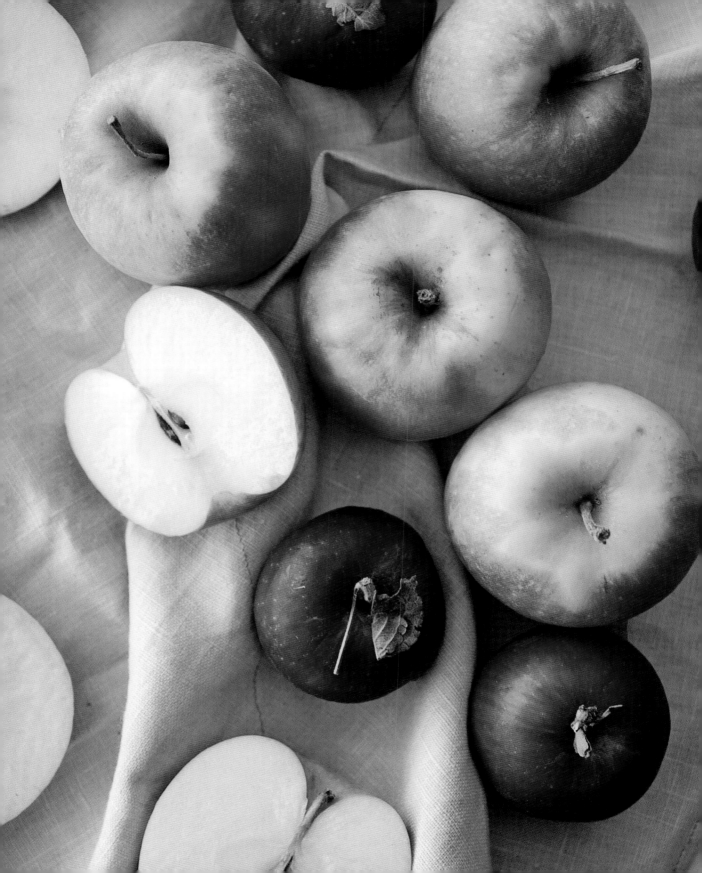

MARSHMALLOWS

Happiness is a homemade marshmallow nestled in a cup of steaming hot cocoa. Or actually, happiness is about one minute later, when the marshmallow starts to melt, slowly enveloping the chocolate in a blanket of white sweetness. Of course, it's easiest to reach into a bag and pop a jet-puffed marshmallow on top of your cup, but if you have twenty minutes, making marshmallows from scratch really makes a difference. Not only is the texture much more tender, but you can also add any flavor you please. And you can make a super-clean, refined-sugar-free version!

MAKES 16 LARGE MARSHMALLOWS

Arrowroot powder for coating

3 tablespoons gelatin powder

1 cup maple syrup

1 tablespoon vanilla extract

¼ teaspoon Himalayan pink salt

1. Line an 8 × 8-inch square pan with parchment paper, and lightly dust the parchment with sifted arrowroot powder. This will prevent the marshmallows from sticking.

2. Pour ½ cup hot water into the bowl of a stand mixer fitted with the whisk attachment. Sprinkle the gelatin on top to soften, stirring gently to fully dissolve it.

3. In a medium saucepan over medium heat, combine another ½ cup water, the maple syrup, vanilla, and salt. Bring the mixture to a simmer and cook, using a candy thermometer to monitor the temperature, until it reaches the soft-ball stage at 240°F. Careful! This happens quickly, so keep a close watch once the syrup reaches 220°F.

4. With the mixer on medium-high speed, blend the gelatin mixture. Slowly pour in the syrup and continue to beat for about 10 minutes, until the steam disappears and soft peaks form. The mixture will become white and super fluffy.

5. Immediately pour the mixture into the prepared pan and allow to set at room temperature for about 4 hours. Sift a light coating of arrowroot powder over the pan, coat a chef's knife with arrowroot powder, and cut the marshmallows into squares. Lightly toss the marshmallows in the pan to evenly coat with arrowroot powder to ensure they do not stick to each other. Lightly dust off excess arrowroot and store in an airtight container at room temperature. They'll keep for up to 1 week, but are best within the first day or so.

Note

To make vegan marshmallows, use soy gelatin powder.

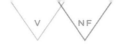

APPLESAUCE

Especially in vegan baking, applesauce is an important ingredient to have in your arsenal. It can add moisture and sweetness to almost any recipe, and can even take on some of the binding properties of eggs. We make our own at home, and love taking advantage of the farmer's market with its seasonal varieties of heirloom apples.

MAKES 4 CUPS

3 pounds apples, peeled, cored, and sliced

Juice of 1 lemon

2 cinnamon sticks

Pinch of Himalayan pink salt

Honey or maple syrup to taste

Ground cinnamon

1. Place the apples, lemon juice, cinnamon sticks, salt, and ½ cup water in a slow cooker and cook on low for about 4 to 6 hours until thick and jammy.

Alternatively, place the apples, lemon juice, cinnamon sticks, and salt in a large saucepan with enough water to barely cover, and simmer for about 50 minutes. The apples should be completely tender and barely golden brown.

2. Let the applesauce cool to room temperature. Remove the cinnamon sticks and transfer to a blender. Pulse the applesauce until it reaches your preferred consistency. Add a little honey or maple syrup for extra sweetness, and serve with a sprinkling of ground cinnamon on top. Refrigerate in a sealed jar for up to 2 weeks.

COCONUT WHIPPED CREAM

Without a doubt, the most frustrating thing to prepare in our bakery is coconut whipped cream. You do everything right, and yet you're staring down into a bowl of goop with a naked cake waiting impatiently on the table to be iced. After one too many restless nights worrying about whether the coconut cream would set, we figured out some workarounds to add stability and guarantee perfect coconut whipped cream, every single time.

First, be sure your coconut milk is left untouched in the coldest part of your fridge (but above 40°F to avoid freezing) at least overnight. (As long as possible is even better. Right after we come home from the market, the can of coconut milk goes straight into the fridge and lives there until we need to use it.) This gives the thick, white cream a chance to rise to the top and settle, making it easy to separate the cream from the clear, liquid coconut water. Second, whip still-solid coconut cream until completely smooth, but no further. This sounds counterintuitive, but if you overwhip the coconut cream, it will soften and become liquid. Once it's whipped to soft or stiff peaks, you can use it as is, or pop it in the fridge overnight for a super-stable cream to fill cakes.

MAKES 2 CUPS

Two 13.5-ounce cans full-fat coconut milk, refrigerated overnight

2 tablespoons maple syrup

1 tablespoon vanilla extract

1. Remove the solid coconut cream that has risen to the top of the can, and spoon it into a stand mixer fitted with the whisk attachment. Beat the coconut cream on high speed until it begins to thicken and peaks form. The remaining coconut water can be added, a teaspoon at a time, if the whipped cream is too thick. Otherwise, discard it.

2. Using a rubber spatula, slowly fold in the maple syrup and vanilla. Transfer the whipped cream to a metal or glass bowl, cover, and refrigerate until ready to use.

Notes

For filling cakes, we like to chill the coconut whipped cream in the fridge overnight, covered. This will stiffen the cream and make it stronger for holding layers of cake together. However, it becomes more difficult to style the cream on top of the cake, so we tend to do this only for the filling between cake layers.

The brand of coconut milk you purchase (see page 249) is not the only thing that can affect the final outcome. If coconut milk has accidentally been frozen or overheated, it can struggle to separate properly. For this reason, we recommend your not ordering coconut milk online, but buying it from a store familiar with storing the product properly, like Whole Foods.

CHAI COCONUT WHIPPED CREAM

WHILE PROCESSING, ADD:

¼ teaspoon ground cinnamon

¼ teaspoon ground ginger

⅛ teaspoon ground cloves

⅛ teaspoon ground cardamom

ESPRESSO COCONUT WHIPPED CREAM

2 teaspoons espresso powder

¼ teaspoon Himalayan pink salt

Combine the espresso and salt with 2 tablespoons hot water. Stir together and let cool. Fold into the coconut whipped cream.

LEMON LAVENDER COCONUT WHIPPED CREAM

WHILE PROCESSING, ADD:

1 teaspoon grated lemon zest

¼ teaspoon ground lavender

GRAPEFRUIT COCONUT WHIPPED CREAM

WHILE PROCESSING, ADD:

2 tablespoons grated grapefruit zest

Additional 2 tablespoons raw honey

CINNAMON-GINGER COCONUT WHIPPED CREAM

WHILE PROCESSING, ADD:

1 teaspoon ground cinnamon

Ginger syrup from Candied Ginger Syrup (page 221) in place of maple syrup

LIME COCONUT WHIPPED CREAM

WHILE PROCESSING, ADD:

Grated zest of 1 lime

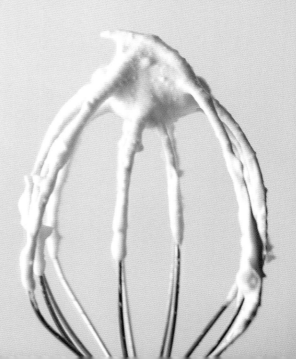

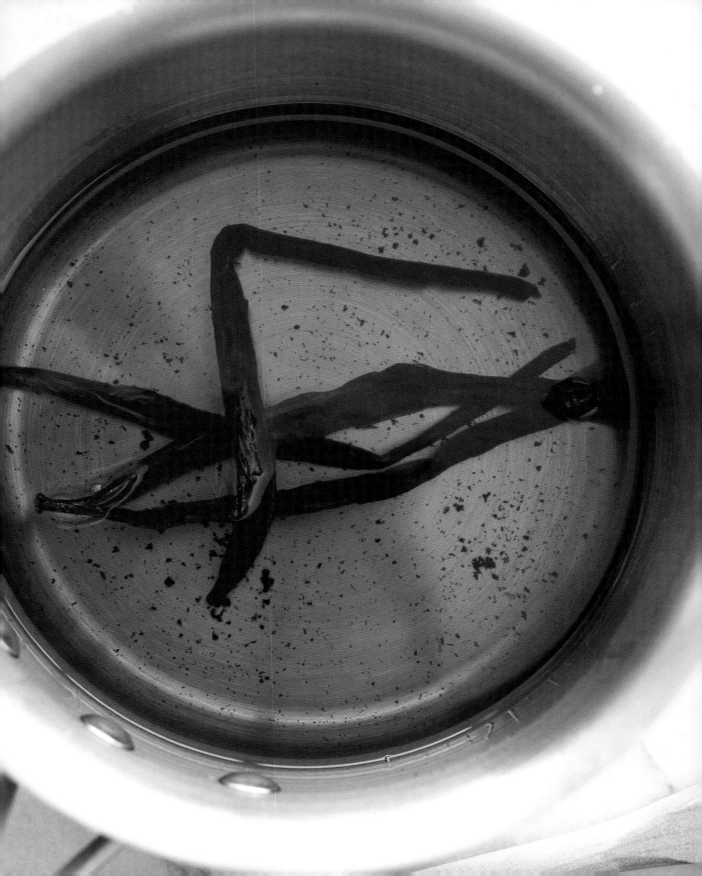

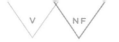

VANILLA EXTRACT

Our grain-free vanilla extract has been the surprise star of our line of pantry ingredients. When we first started baking grain-free, vanilla extract was impossible to find at the store since most base alcohols come from grains or refined starches with gluten. So what's a girl to do? We quickly zeroed in on tequila (we may or may not have had margaritas in our hands at the time) and started brewing our own extract for baking. The best part? It's easy to make, gets better with time, and even makes a beautiful gift.

MAKES 2 CUPS

2 cups tequila blanco	1 tablespoon vanilla bean powder (see page 249) or 2 whole vanilla beans, seeds scraped

1. Pour the tequila into a large Mason jar with a tight-fitting lid.

2. Add the vanilla bean powder or seeds and pods to the jar. Tighten the lid, shake the contents to blend everything together, and put the jar in a dark place, as light can cause organic compounds to break down (it's one of the reasons extracts and good olive oil are sold in dark bottles).

3. Each day, give the vanilla extract a shake. It will be ready to use after about 6 weeks. We run out of the extract before ever hitting an expiration date, but if stored in a cool, dry place with the bottle securely sealed, it should last indefinitely.

BAKING POWDER

This is an incredibly simple pantry staple, and a DIY version probably seems unnecessary. However, conventional baking powders can have additives like aluminum, so we prefer to make our own clean, natural version. Once you whip this up yourself, you'll always have a batch ready for baking.

MAKES ¾ CUP

½ cup cream of tartar, sifted	¼ cup baking soda, sifted

Sift together the cream of tartar and baking soda into a small jar. Tighten the lid and keep in a cool, dry place.

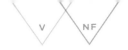

VEGAN EGGS

Every now and then we get vegan orders for our cakes, which, when you consider all of the other things *not* in our cakes, makes for a baking challenge. Luckily, there are some fabulous vegan binder replacements. Ground flaxseed creates a nice gooey texture and has a lovely nutty flavor. Chia seed has a similar effect but with greater health benefits, such as impressive amounts of omega-3 essential fatty acids, protein, and fiber per gram. Psyllium husk powder is great when you need something with super-binding or super-rising qualities, such as for custards or quick breads, or are making a lighter-colored cake. (It's also used as a supplement to improve and speed up digestion.)

For all of these replacements, just mix with hot water and add them to the recipe when you would add a regular egg. (Note that flax and chia seed needs to "gel" in the refrigerator for a few minutes.) Scale up the amounts as needed for the number of eggs desired.

**EACH VEGAN EGG REPLACES
1 LARGE CHICKEN EGG**

FOR 1 FLAXSEED EGG

Grind 1 tablespoon flaxseed in a spice grinder (or use flaxseed meal) and stir into 3 tablespoons hot water. Set for 15 minutes in the fridge before using.

FOR 1 CHIA SEED EGG

Grind 1 tablespoon chia seed in a spice grinder and stir into 3 tablespoons hot water. Set for 5 minutes in the fridge before using.

FOR 1 PSYLLIUM EGG

Stir 1 tablespoon psyllium husk powder into ¼ cup hot water. Use immediately.

Note

Vegan eggs do not work well with coconut flour, as it requires so much additional moisture. If you must swap regular eggs for vegan eggs, and are using coconut flour, add an additional 2 tablespoons of coconut milk for each vegan egg.

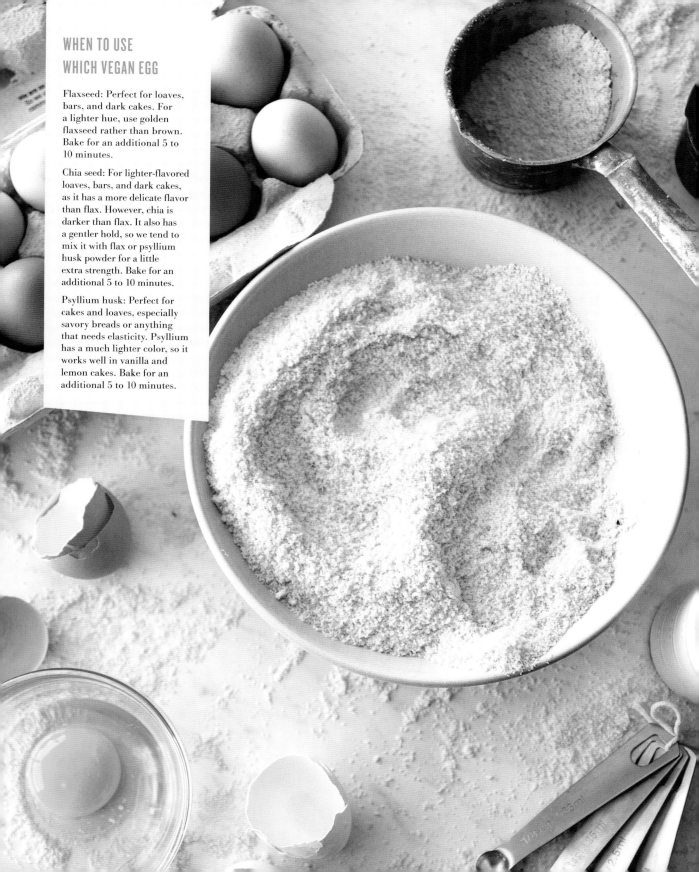

WHEN TO USE WHICH VEGAN EGG

Flaxseed: Perfect for loaves, bars, and dark cakes. For a lighter hue, use golden flaxseed rather than brown. Bake for an additional 5 to 10 minutes.

Chia seed: For lighter-flavored loaves, bars, and dark cakes, as it has a more delicate flavor than flax. However, chia is darker than flax. It also has a gentler hold, so we tend to mix it with flax or psyllium husk powder for a little extra strength. Bake for an additional 5 to 10 minutes.

Psyllium husk: Perfect for cakes and loaves, especially savory breads or anything that needs elasticity. Psyllium has a much lighter color, so it works well in vanilla and lemon cakes. Bake for an additional 5 to 10 minutes.

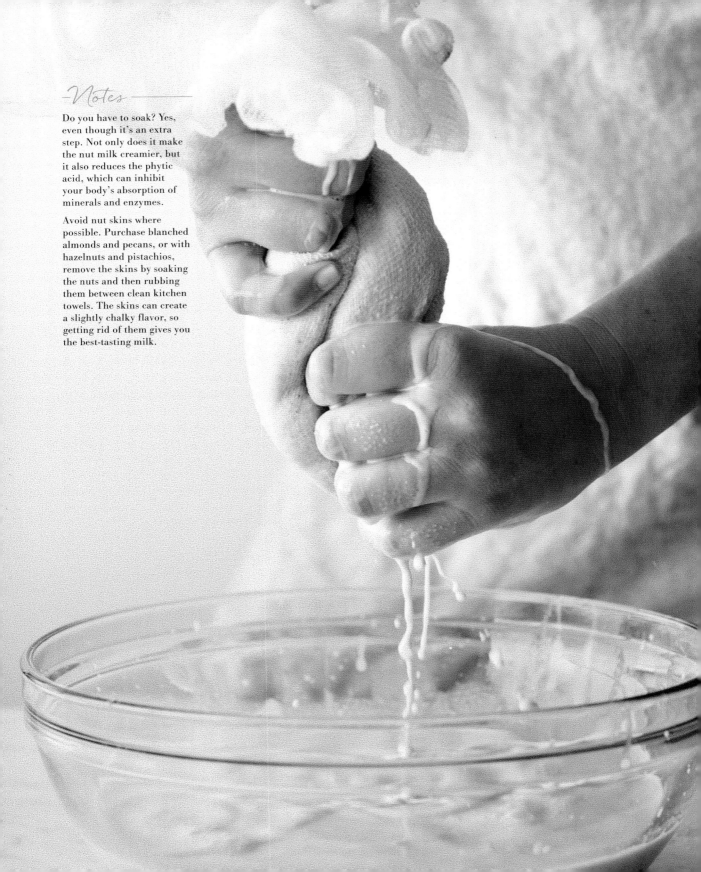

Notes

Do you have to soak? Yes, even though it's an extra step. Not only does it make the nut milk creamier, but it also reduces the phytic acid, which can inhibit your body's absorption of minerals and enzymes.

Avoid nut skins where possible. Purchase blanched almonds and pecans, or with hazelnuts and pistachios, remove the skins by soaking the nuts and then rubbing them between clean kitchen towels. The skins can create a slightly chalky flavor, so getting rid of them gives you the best-tasting milk.

ALMOND MILK

We love almond milk. In our coffee, in our cereal, in our cakes, or just in a glass, we sip, gulp, and practically luxuriate in it. Homemade almond milk has a rich, velvety texture that's unlike anything available in the store, plus you know exactly what's in it. (Store-bought versions can include binders and emulsifiers, and tend to be much thinner in texture.) Better yet, you can add flavoring to get it exactly how you like it. This recipe is our simplest version, but we love almond milk mixed with matcha, rose water, or turmeric for something different. You can also make milk from cashews, Brazil nuts, hazelnuts, and walnuts! Just soak and process them the same way.

MAKES 2 QUARTS

4 cups raw almonds

2 tablespoons date paste, store-bought or homemade (page 42)

1 teaspoon vanilla extract

Pinch of Himalayan pink salt

1. Place the almonds in a large bowl and cover completely with water. Refrigerate for at least 8 hours.

2. Drain the almonds and put them in a blender. Working in batches as needed, add 10 cups water, the date paste, vanilla, and salt. Blend on high for about 2 minutes, until the mixture starts to look creamy.

3. Strain the mixture through a cheesecloth or nut-milk bag, squeezing the almond milk into a large bowl. Transfer to a jar and tighten the lid. Reserve the leftover almond meal in the refrigerator to make almond flour (recipe follows), if desired. The almond milk will keep for 3 to 5 days in the fridge. You can tell it's no longer good when it smells sour, just like regular milk.

ALMOND FLOUR

When our bakery launched, California was in the middle of a historic drought. Almond prices skyrocketed, and the idea of using an ingredient so drought-intolerant weighed on us as we were baking our first cakes. Luckily, we came up with a sustainable solution. We bought the almond meal left over from milk production and dehydrated it to make our own flour. The residual meal is quite dry, as the fat has been stripped from the almonds, so in our recipes, we like to use a 50/50 mix of homemade and store-bought almond flour.

MAKES 4 CUPS

8 cups almond meal, reserved from preceding almond milk recipe

1. Place the almond meal on the trays of a dehydrator. Spread the meal evenly throughout the tray, making sure not to overcrowd. Dehydrate at 110°F for 12 hours. If you don't have a dehydrator, you can do this overnight in the oven. Spread the meal evenly over 2 rimmed baking sheets. Turn your oven to the lowest setting (200°F or lower) and leave the door cracked slightly.

2. Once the meal is completely dry, transfer it to a blender. Pulse on high for about 8 seconds, or until the meal looks like flour. Keep a close watch, being careful not to overblend, which would lead to almond butter. Store in an airtight container at room temperature. The almond flour will turn if there is residual moisture or it gets wet; otherwise, it lasts as long as any store-bought grain-free flour.

Note

Fresh almond meal that is still wet freezes beautifully, which is a good thing, because wet almond meal has a shelf life of only about 18 hours. In the freezer it can last for several months.

CASHEW PUREE or BUTTER

Cashew puree, also known as cashew butter, is a vegan culinary building block. It can make a soup creamy and rich, become cheese if agitated correctly, or whip into a beautiful frosting—all while retaining a delicate, simple flavor that nestles comfortably into the background. We fold it into our recipes for extra moisture and a velvety, rich texture, or use it as the base for a light and simple frosting.

MAKES 2 CUPS

4 cups raw cashews	Pinch of Himalayan pink salt

I. Place the cashews in a large bowl and cover completely with water. Refrigerate for at least 8 hours.

2. Drain the cashews and dry them off completely with a kitchen towel. Place the cashews and salt in a high-powered blender and puree until creamy.

3. Transfer the puree to a glass jar, tighten the lid, and refrigerate for up to 2 months.

ALMOND BUTTER

Almond butter is one of the cornerstone ingredients at Sweet Laurel. More than just a favorite snack swiped across a piece of toast, it's the base for our ganache frosting and our vegan caramel. Just like almond milk, it's incredibly versatile and begs for experimentation. We've shared some of our favorite variations. Our base almond butter is roasted to bring out the nuts' oils, but you can skip this step to keep it raw.

MAKES 1½ CUPS

3 cups raw almonds

I. Place the almonds in a large bowl and cover completely with water. Refrigerate for at least 8 hours. Drain and dry off completely with a kitchen towel.

2. Preheat the oven to 400°F.

3. Spread the almonds on a baking sheet and roast for about 7 minutes. You should be able to smell them roasting.

4. Transfer the almonds to a food processor or high-powered blender and allow to process for about 30 minutes, stopping and scraping down the sides with a rubber spatula periodically. The almond butter is ready when smooth and creamy—this takes more time than you'd expect, so be patient!

5. Transfer the almond butter to a glass jar, tighten the lid, and refrigerate for up to 2 months.

HONEY ALMOND BUTTER

WHILE PROCESSING, ADD:

2 tablespoons raw honey

¼ teaspoon
Himalayan pink salt

CINNAMON ALMOND BUTTER

WHILE PROCESSING, ADD:

1 teaspoon
ground cinnamon

1 tablespoon maple syrup

¼ teaspoon
Himalayan pink salt

CHOCOLATE SPICE ALMOND BUTTER

WHILE PROCESSING, ADD:

¼ cup 100% cacao
unsweetened baking
chocolate, melted

½ teaspoon
ground cinnamon

3 tablespoons maple
syrup

¼ teaspoon cayenne

¼ teaspoon
Himalayan pink salt

CHAI ALMOND BUTTER

WHILE PROCESSING, ADD:

1 teaspoon ground ginger

½ teaspoon
ground cardamom

¼ teaspoon
ground cinnamon

⅛ teaspoon
ground cloves

3 tablespoons raw honey

¼ teaspoon
Himalayan pink salt

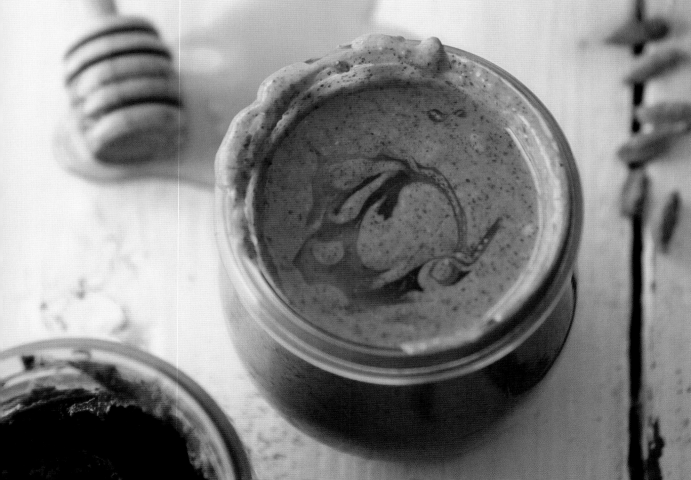

COCONUT
YOGURT

We have a problem. A coconut yogurt problem. Meaning, we're obsessed with its creamy but sharp deliciousness. After almost purchasing a $40 quart of coconut yogurt at our local health food store, we decided things had gotten out of hand, and it was time to make our own. You can use a yogurt maker or just let it ferment in your oven, and you'll get a delicious ingredient to enjoy with fruit for breakfast or as a buttermilk replacement in pancakes, waffles, and more. You can also make an unsweetened version of this yogurt by leaving out the vanilla extract and maple syrup. Laurel loves her unsweetened coco yogurt!

MAKES 2 CUPS

Two 13.5-ounce cans full-fat coconut milk, refrigerated overnight

2 probiotic capsules (see page 249)

½ teaspoon raw honey or maple syrup

½ teaspoon vanilla extract, optional

1. Remove the solid coconut cream that has risen to the top of the cans and spoon it into a large, sterilized glass jar, leaving just enough room to add the additional ingredients.

2. Open the probiotic capsules and stir the contents into the coconut cream along with the honey or maple syrup and the vanilla, if using. Loosely screw on the lid.

3. Place the jar in a dehydrator set to 110°F for 18 to 24 hours. If you don't have a dehydrator, place the jar in your oven with the light on. The light emits a bit of heat, making the oven a good place for fermentation. After the fermenting period, refrigerate the yogurt until ready to use, for up to 1 week.

VEGAN
CARAMEL

We believe our early success has a lot to do with this recipe. There have been vegan caramel super fans since day one (seriously, one guy has a weekly order), and once you try it, you'll know why. You'll see it pop up in a few recipes in this cookbook, but we won't judge if you eat this straight out of the jar with a spoon! Our favorite way of serving it is on top of sliced bananas, or with a piece of dark chocolate. You can buy ours at sweetlaurel.com, but here's our secret recipe.

MAKES ½ CUP

¼ cup almond or cashew butter or puree, store-bought or homemade (page 38)

¼ cup maple syrup

2 tablespoons coconut oil, melted

1 or 2 fresh dates, pitted

1 teaspoon vanilla extract

Pinch of Himalayan pink salt

1. Place all of the ingredients in a blender or food processor and puree until smooth.

2. Transfer the caramel to a glass jar and place in the refrigerator to chill. The caramel will stiffen up in the refrigerator, so if your recipe calls for it to be spreadable, let the caramel sit at room temperature for 30 minutes to an hour, and give it a good stir before using. The caramel will keep for about 1 month, refrigerated.

Note

If you want a thinner sauce to drizzle on top of a dessert, just add another 2 tablespoons maple syrup. For a denser, caramel candy texture, add 2 more dates. For spreading on cake layers, add 2 more tablespoons almond or cashew butter.

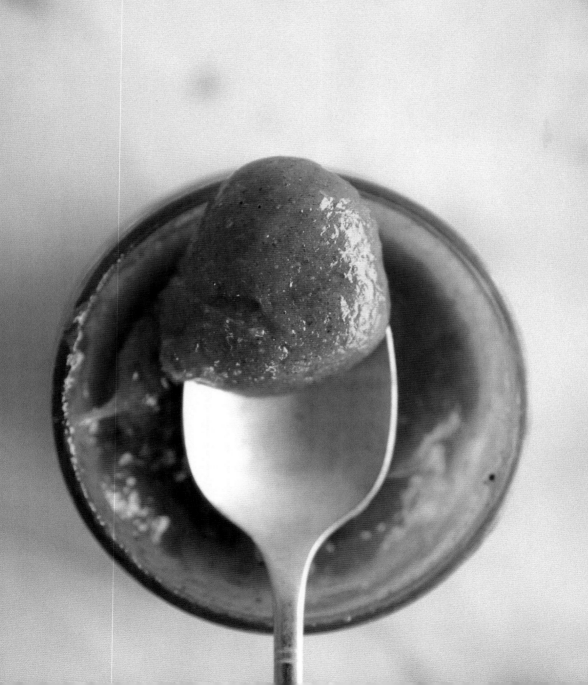

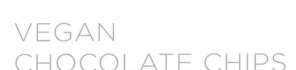

VEGAN CHOCOLATE CHIPS

We both keep a flashlight under our bed and these chocolate chips in the pantry, just in case of emergencies. Making your own chocolate chips sounds fussy, but these require just three ingredients, are easy to make, and are completely customizable.

MAKES 1 CUP

4 ounces 100% cacao unsweetened baking chocolate, roughly chopped

1 tablespoon coconut oil, solid

2 to 3 tablespoons maple syrup

1. Line a large, rimmed baking sheet with parchment paper.

2. Melt the cacao and coconut oil in a medium saucepan over very low heat, stirring constantly. It's easy to burn chocolate, so be sure to watch the pot and keep the mixture moving.

3. When the mixture is almost completely melted, remove the pan from the heat. Slowly stir in the maple syrup. For bittersweet chocolate chips, add 2 tablespoons syrup; for sweeter, add 3 tablespoons. Pour the mixture onto the baking sheet and use a rubber spatula to spread it evenly. Place the baking sheet in the freezer for at least 30 minutes, or until the chocolate is matte and hard.

4. Once the chocolate has hardened completely, remove it from the baking sheet and chop it into ¼- to ½-inch-wide pieces. Stored in an airtight container, the chocolate chips will keep in the freezer or refrigerator for at least 2 months.

Note

We keep our Vegan Chocolate Chips in the freezer, which not only extends their shelf life, but also means they won't soften and stick together.

DATE PASTE

Date paste is one of our favorite secret ingredients. Put a piece in almond milk for a creamier, richer texture; mix it with cacao powder to make instant truffles; or just serve it on a cheese board—it's ridiculously versatile. Our favorite date company actually makes its paste using a meat grinder, to get an even consistency. If you're planning on doing quite a bit of refined-sugar-free cooking, having a pound of date paste in your fridge, kept the way you would a pound of butter, is a great idea. It will always be ready and convenient to use.

MAKES 1 CUP

20 Medjool dates, pitted

1. Place the dates in a medium bowl, cover with hot water, and soak for about 5 minutes, until very tender and falling apart when squeezed between your thumb and forefinger. If the dates are extra tough, you may need to soak them longer.

2. Strain the dates and place them in a blender or food processor. Pulse until the dates are blended but not completely smooth.

3. Transfer the date paste to a sealed glass jar or wrap tightly in plastic wrap; refrigerate for up to 3 months.

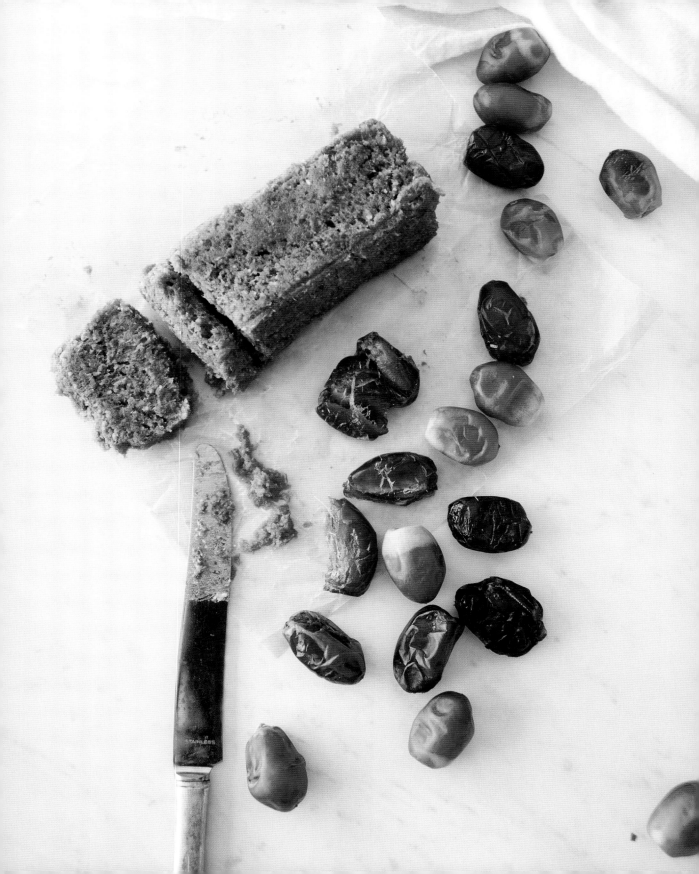

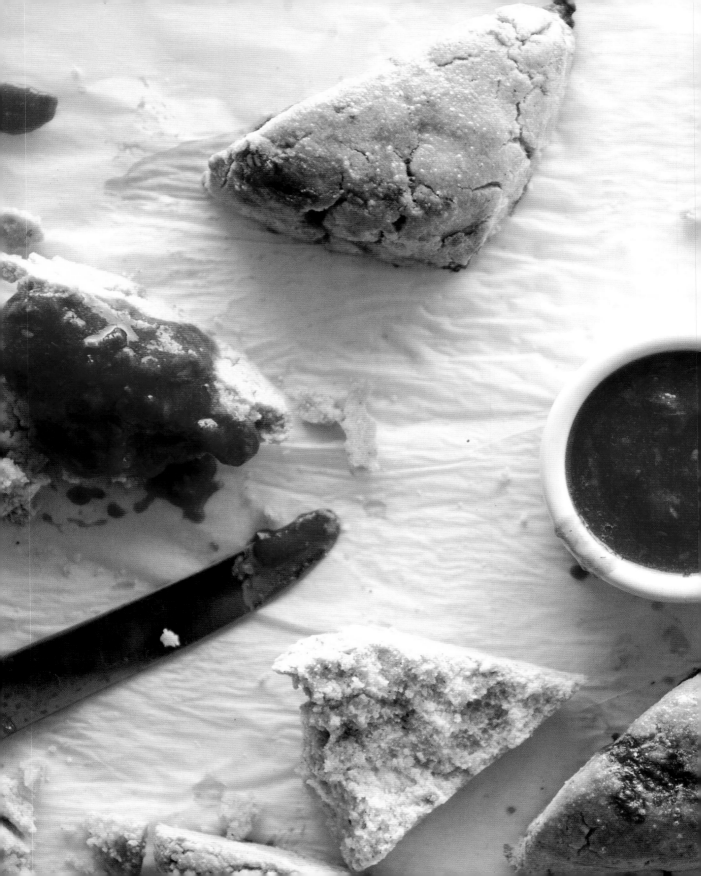

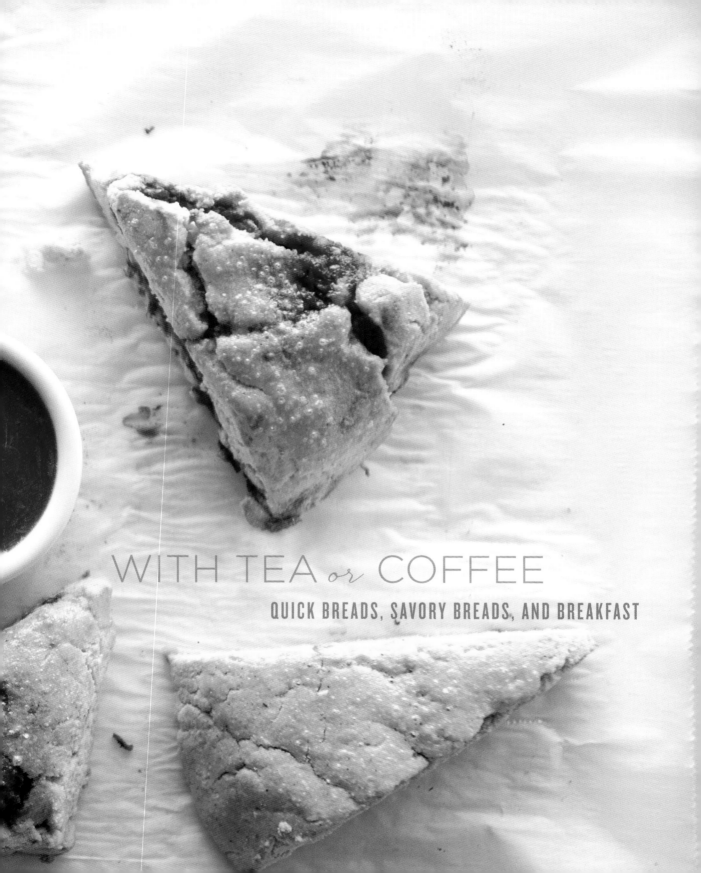

WITH TEA *or* COFFEE

QUICK BREADS, SAVORY BREADS, AND BREAKFAST

MOTHER'S SCONES

Both of us grew up sipping from teacups and brushing crumbs off our skirts. Our mothers love afternoon tea, and at the beginning of our friendship, we'd spend hours chatting over a pot. Even today, we'll pick up vintage porcelain cups and saucers for each other from flea markets. Part of any good afternoon tea is, of course, scones. We like our scones the old-fashioned, British way: not too sweet, with a tender, not-too-dense crumb. These should be served with plenty of coconut whipped cream, jam, and, of course, conversation.

MAKES 6 SCONES

1½ cups almond flour

¼ cup coconut flour

1 tablespoon baking powder

¼ teaspoon Himalayan pink salt

3 tablespoons maple syrup

¾ cup coconut yogurt, store-bought or homemade (page 40), fully chilled

1 tablespoon vanilla extract

Optional fillings: chocolate chips, blueberries, grated orange zest

Berry Jam Filling (page 208) and Coconut Whipped Cream (page 30), for serving

1. Preheat the oven to 350°F. Line a baking sheet with parchment paper.

2. Whisk together the flours, baking powder, and salt in a medium bowl. In a large bowl, combine the maple syrup, coconut yogurt, and vanilla. A little at a time, add the dry ingredients to the wet, stirring until a dough comes together. Fold in any desired fillings.

3. Pat the dough into a ball. Press down to form a circle about 2 inches thick. Using a chef's knife, cut the circle into 6 triangles. Spread the wedges out on the baking sheet and bake for 10 to 15 minutes, until barely golden on the top and golden on the bottom.

4. Serve the scones warm or at room temperature with berry jam and coconut whipped cream alongside. Store in a sealed container at room temperature for up to 3 days, warming in a low oven before serving, if desired.

MOCHA CHIP MUFFINS

We love our coffee at Sweet Laurel, mostly because it prompts the question, "What cake would you like with it?" But for this recipe, we combine the cake and coffee into one delicious muffin. The touch of cacao brings out the freshly ground espresso, and the sprinkling of cinnamon gives the muffin a *café de olla* vibe.

MAKES 9 MUFFINS

2½ cups almond flour

½ teaspoon baking soda

½ teaspoon Himalayan pink salt

1 tablespoon finely ground espresso

1 tablespoon 100% unsweetened cacao powder

¼ teaspoon ground cinnamon

½ cup maple syrup

2 large eggs

¼ cup coconut oil, melted

1 tablespoon vanilla extract

1 cup vegan chocolate chips, store-bought or homemade (page 42)

1. Preheat the oven to 350°F. Line 9 muffin cups with paper liners.

2. In a large bowl, whisk together the flour, baking soda, salt, espresso, cacao powder, and cinnamon. In a medium bowl, whisk the maple syrup, eggs, coconut oil, and vanilla. A little at a time, add the dry ingredients to the wet, stirring until a batter forms. Fold in the chocolate chips.

3. Divide the batter among the lined muffin cups, filling each three-fourths of the way. Bake for 20 to 25 minutes, or until a toothpick inserted into the center comes out clean. Remove the muffins from the tin, set on a rack, and allow to cool completely. Store in a sealed container at room temperature for up to 3 days for ideal freshness or freeze for up to 2 months. Defrost before reheating in a low oven.

DOUBLE CHOCOLATE MUFFINS

Is it cheating to call these muffins when they're basically mini chocolate cakes? We think they get a pass, since one of these little guys has 10 grams of protein, making it a pretty reasonable breakfast choice. For extra decadence, we drizzle the muffins with melted cacao and serve them with a cup of coffee with almond milk. Can mornings get any better than that?

MAKES 9 MUFFINS

2½ cups almond flour

¼ cup 100% unsweetened cacao powder

1 teaspoon baking soda

½ teaspoon Himalayan pink salt

¾ cup maple syrup

2 large eggs

1 tablespoon vanilla extract

1 cup vegan chocolate chips, store-bought or homemade (page 42)

1. Preheat the oven to 350°F. Line 9 muffin cups with paper liners.

2. In a large bowl, whisk together the almond flour, cacao powder, baking soda, and salt. In a separate bowl, combine the maple syrup, eggs, and vanilla. A little at a time, add the dry ingredients to the wet, stirring until a batter forms. Fold in ½ cup of the chocolate chips.

3. Divide the batter among the 9 lined muffin cups, filling each three-fourths of the way. Bake for 20 to 25 minutes, until a toothpick inserted into the center comes out clean. Remove the muffins from the tin, set on a rack, and allow to cool completely.

4. To make the chocolate drizzle, melt the remaining chocolate chips in a glass bowl, either for 10 seconds in a microwave or over a pot of boiling water (see Note). Use a spoon to drizzle the melted chocolate over each muffin. Let the drizzle set, then serve. Store in a sealed container at room temperature for up to 3 days for ideal freshness or freeze for up to 2 months. Defrost before reheating in a low oven.

───── *Note* ─────

Chocolate is notorious for burning over direct heat, so to melt it, use a double boiler, or create one: Just place the chocolate in a glass or metal bowl set over a pot of simmering water, being sure the bottom of the bowl is at least an inch above the water.

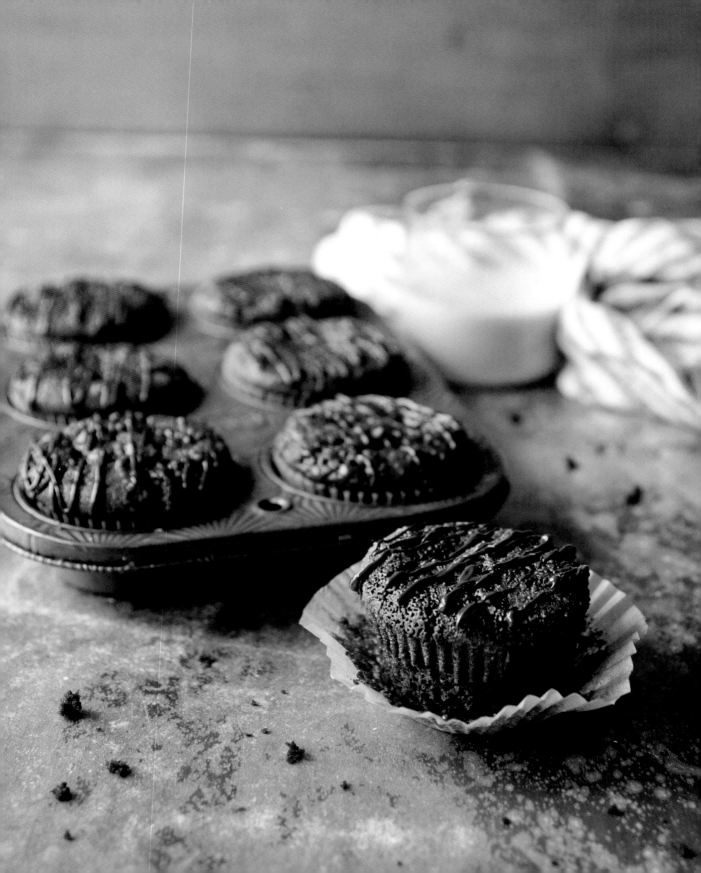

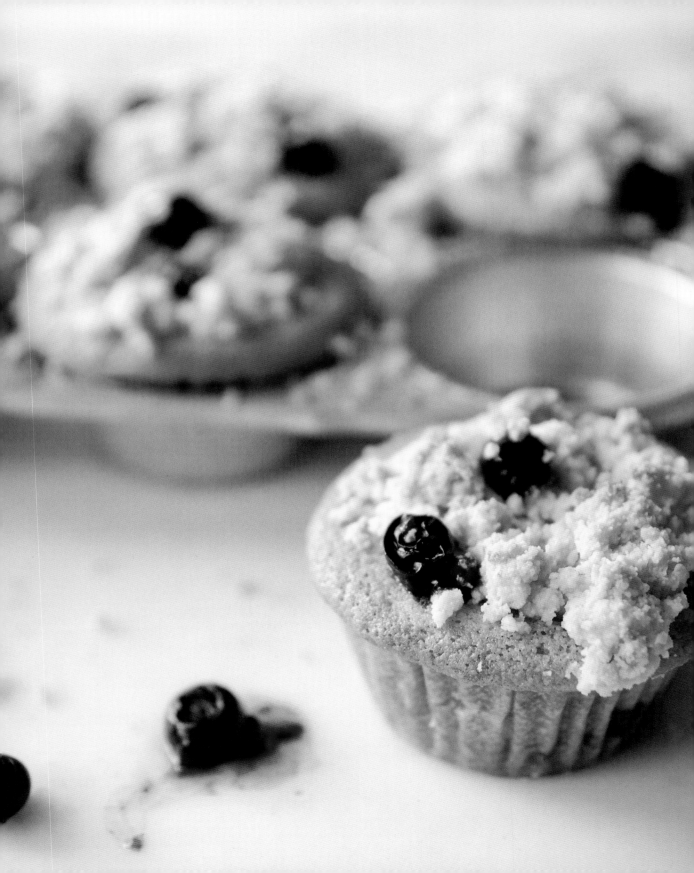

BLUEBERRY STREUSEL MUFFINS

After the chocolate cake that launched our bakery (see page 167), blueberry bread was the second baked good to emerge from our ovens. There's just something so satisfying about blueberry-studded cake punctuated with flecks of lemon zest. For breakfast, we changed the bread into a muffin and added a crunchy and sweet streusel on top. With a cup of coffee, it makes for the perfect morning.

MAKES 8 MUFFINS

FOR THE STREUSEL

½ cup almond flour

1 tablespoon coconut oil, melted

1 tablespoon maple syrup

FOR THE MUFFINS

2½ cups almond flour

¾ teaspoon baking soda

¼ teaspoon Himalayan pink salt

4 large eggs, at room temperature

⅓ cup coconut oil, melted

⅔ cup maple syrup

1½ teaspoons grated lemon zest, packed

1 tablespoon fresh lemon juice

2 tablespoons vanilla extract

4 ounces blueberries

1. Preheat the oven to 350°F. Line a baking sheet with parchment paper. Line 8 muffin cups with paper liners.

2. **MAKE THE STREUSEL:** In a small bowl, whisk together the flour, oil, and maple syrup until the mixture comes together. Crumble onto the baking sheet and bake for 20 minutes, or until the streusel begins to crisp up. Remove and set aside, but keep the oven on at 350°F.

3. **MAKE THE MUFFINS:** In a large bowl, whisk together the flour, baking soda, and salt. In a separate bowl, combine the eggs, coconut oil, maple syrup, lemon zest and juice, and vanilla. A little at a time, add the dry ingredients to the wet, stirring until a smooth batter forms.

4. Divide the batter among the 8 lined muffin cups, filling each three-fourths of the way. Top each muffin with a few blueberries and lightly swirl them into the batter with a spoon. Sprinkle the streusel topping over the muffins.

5. Bake for about 25 minutes, until the streusel is golden brown. Remove the muffins from the tin, set on a rack, and allow to cool completely. Store for up to 5 days in a sealed container, or for up to 2 months in the freezer. Defrost before reheating in a low oven.

----- *Note* -----

Blueberry is a classic, but you can swap in any berries or stone fruit in this recipe. If the fruit is very juicy or watery, like strawberries, bake for an extra 5 minutes.

FALL-IN-LOVE BANANA BREAD

When Laurel met the man who would become her husband, she had an inexplicable desire to make him banana bread on their second date. Where this urge came from, she'll never know, but thank goodness it did. As it turns out, banana bread was Nick's childhood favorite. By the time he finished his first bite, he knew he was going to marry her. Years later they made banana bread for each guest at their wedding, all four hundred of them! Truly, this recipe is a labor of love.

MAKES TWO 9 × 5-INCH LOAVES

⅓ cup coconut oil, melted

2 cups mashed banana (about 4 to 6 ripe bananas)

⅔ cup maple syrup

2 large eggs

1 teaspoon vanilla extract

2 cups almond flour

½ teaspoon baking soda

½ teaspoon Himalayan pink salt

½ cup vegan chocolate chips, store-bought or homemade (page 42)

2 bananas, halved lengthwise

1. Preheat the oven to 350°F. Line two 9 × 5-inch loaf pans with parchment paper, letting the paper hang over the sides for easy removal, or grease the pans with coconut oil.

2. In a large bowl, beat together the coconut oil, mashed banana, maple syrup, eggs, and vanilla with a hand mixer. In a medium bowl, whisk the flour, baking soda, and salt. A little at a time, add the dry ingredients to the wet and beat until a batter forms. Fold in the chocolate chips.

3. Divide the batter between the prepared loaf pans. Arrange 2 banana halves on top of each loaf and gently press them into the batter. Bake for 40 to 45 minutes, until a toothpick inserted into the center of the loaves comes out clean. Remove the bread from the pans, set on a rack, and allow to cool completely before slicing.

CLASSIC SANDWICH BREAD

When Laurel had to rework her diet after her Hashimoto's diagnosis, one of the casualties was her favorite breakfast: toasted whole-wheat bread with almond butter. Most of the gluten-free bread options out there still contain sugar, dairy, fillers, or gums, and the cleaner options were a challenge to toast and get that delicious crunch. So she developed her own! This is the simplest bread we make at Sweet Laurel, and it's a wonderful multipurpose recipe to keep dog-eared. Use it to make sandwiches, crostini, toast, even Thanksgiving stuffing or bread pudding—the dough also freezes perfectly if you want to bake off a bunch at a time.

MAKES TWO 9 × 5-INCH LOAVES

1 cup almond flour

2 teaspoons baking soda

1 teaspoon Himalayan pink salt

2 cups cashew butter (page 38)

4 large eggs, plus 4 large egg whites

¼ cup fresh lemon juice

1. Preheat the oven to 350°F. Line two 9 × 5-inch loaf pans with parchment paper, letting the paper hang over the sides for easy removal, or grease the pans with coconut oil.

2. In a medium bowl, whisk together the flour, baking soda, and salt. In the bowl of a stand mixer fitted with the paddle attachment, blend the cashew butter, eggs, and egg whites on medium speed until smooth. Slowly add the lemon juice on low speed. A little at a time, add the dry ingredients to the mixer and beat until well combined. Transfer the batter to the prepared pans.

3. Bake for 20 to 30 minutes, until a toothpick inserted into the center comes out clean. Remove the bread from the pans, set on a rack, and allow to cool completely before slicing.

CREPES
with LEMON AND HONEY

The crepes we encountered while traveling in France were very different from the ones back home. Presented almost unadorned, with a touch of sugar and melting butter, or a scrape of chocolate hazelnut spread, the crepe is as important as the toppings. So in keeping with that mind-set, we feature our crepes with a drizzle of raw honey, a squeeze of lemon, and some coconut "powdered sugar." It's a lovely mix of bright and sweet, and the perfect simple breakfast.

MAKES 1 DOZEN CREPES

¼ cup coconut flour

6 large eggs

2 tablespoons coconut oil, melted, plus more for greasing the pan

1 cup almond milk

2 tablespoons maple syrup

¼ teaspoon Himalayan pink salt

Shredded Coconut "Powdered Sugar" (page 66), for garnish

1 lemon, halved

Raw honey

1. In a blender, pulse together the flour and eggs. Add the coconut oil, almond milk, maple syrup, and salt and pulse until thoroughly combined.

2. Heat a little coconut oil in a medium sauté pan over medium-low heat.

3. Scoop about 3 tablespoons of the batter onto the skillet and tilt the pan to spread the batter to the edges. It should be quite thin.

4. Cook until small bubbles form on the crepe, then flip and cook the other side, 4 to 5 minutes total. The crepe should be golden brown on both sides. Transfer the crepe to a plate and cover with a kitchen towel to keep warm. If making ahead of time, hold them in a low oven for up to 20 minutes before serving (too much longer in the oven may dry them out). Repeat with the remaining batter, reoiling the pan as necessary.

5. You can roll up the crepes to serve, or enjoy flat on a plate. Garnish with the powdered coconut, a squeeze of lemon juice, and a drizzle of raw honey.

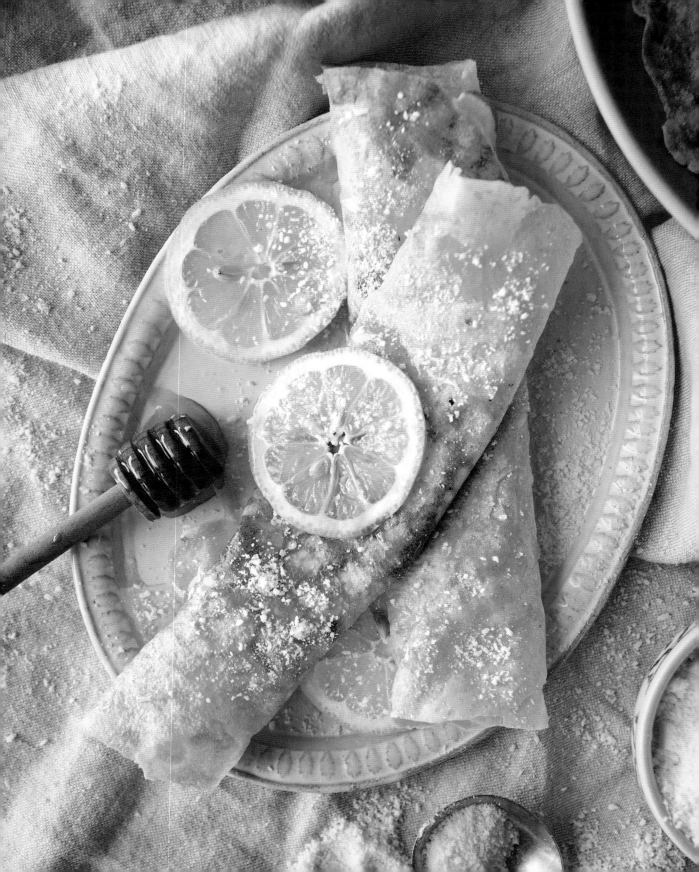

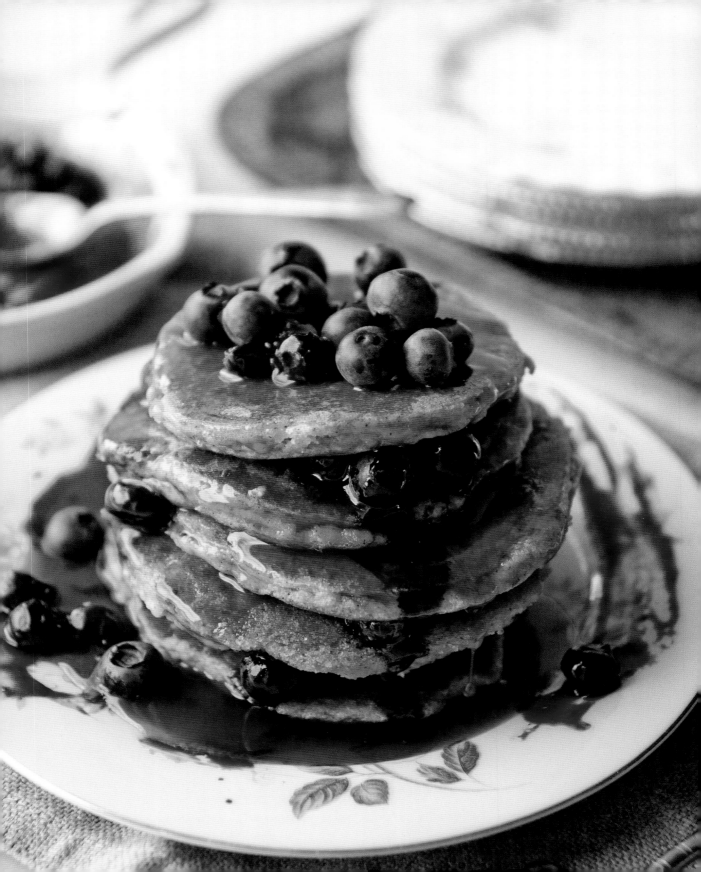

ALMOND PANCAKES
with COCONUT SYRUP

Everyone fantasizes about the perfect breakfast in bed. It comes with a glass of orange juice, a newspaper, and a flower in a bud vase. You're in a kimono with a chic eye mask resting on your forehead—right? This is a universal fantasy? OK, maybe it's just us, but we feel like breakfast in bed should be an indulgent occasion, whatever the reason you're enjoying one. And pancakes seem like the perfect centerpiece for such a morning spread. These are immensely simple, served with fresh blueberries, though we love them with walnuts and chocolate chips, too.

MAKES 10 SMALL PANCAKES

2½ cups almond flour

¾ cup unsweetened applesauce, store-bought or homemade (page 29)

4 large eggs

¾ teaspoon baking powder

½ teaspoon ground cinnamon

½ teaspoon vanilla extract

Coconut oil

Coconut Syrup (recipe follows) and blueberries, for serving

1. Whisk together the flour, applesauce, eggs, baking powder, cinnamon, and vanilla in a large bowl until a batter forms. Be sure to break up any clumps.

2. Set a large skillet over medium heat and melt enough coconut oil to coat the bottom of the pan. Pour about ¼ cup of the pancake batter into the pan, letting it spread out a bit. After about 3 minutes, when bubbles form on the surface, flip the pancake. Cook for 2 to 3 minutes more, until golden brown on the bottom. Repeat with the remaining batter, reoiling the pan as necessary.

3. Serve the pancakes hot with coconut syrup and blueberries on top.

Coconut Syrup

V NF **MAKES 1 CUP**

1 cup maple syrup

1 cup full-fat coconut milk

⅛ teaspoon Himalayan pink salt

1. In a small saucepan, combine all of the ingredients over medium heat. Bring to a boil and then simmer for 5 minutes, or until the mixture is reduced by half and has a syrupy consistency.

2. Pour the syrup into a glass jar and allow to cool slightly. Store any leftovers in the fridge for up to 2 weeks. Gently reheat to loosen the syrup before using.

VANILLA-SCENTED WAFFLES

Fluffy, barely sweet waffles topped with loads of coconut whipped cream and fruit are about as close as you can get to breakfast perfection. Add berries, nuts, chocolate, spices, or whatever else you like to mix it up. You can even remove the vanilla and maple syrup and serve the waffles with eggs and hot sauce.

MAKES 2 TO 4 WAFFLES

⅓ cup full-fat coconut milk

3 tablespoons coconut oil, melted

1 tablespoon maple syrup

2 teaspoons vanilla extract

¼ teaspoon apple cider vinegar

1¼ cups almond flour

1 teaspoon baking powder

¼ teaspoon Himalayan pink salt

3 large eggs

Coconut oil cooking spray, or coconut oil with a pastry brush, for greasing the waffle iron

Fresh fruit and Coconut Whipped Cream (page 30), for serving

1. Preheat your waffle iron according to the manufacturer's instructions.

2. Combine the coconut milk, coconut oil, maple syrup, vanilla, vinegar, flour, baking powder, salt, and eggs in a blender and pulse until a batter forms.

3. Spray the waffle iron with cooking spray (or, if you prefer, carefully coat the iron with melted coconut oil using a pastry brush). Pour a quarter of the batter into the waffle iron, spread with a spatula—the batter will be quite thick—and cook according to the manufacturer's instructions. Repeat with the remaining batter, greasing the iron between each waffle.

4. Serve the waffles hot with fresh fruit and lots of coconut whipped cream.

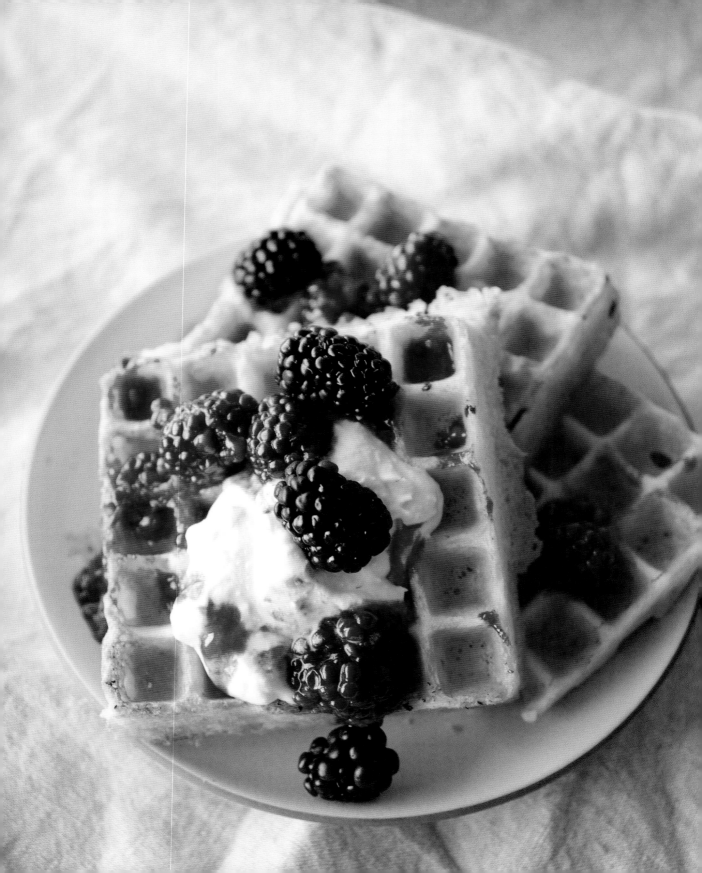

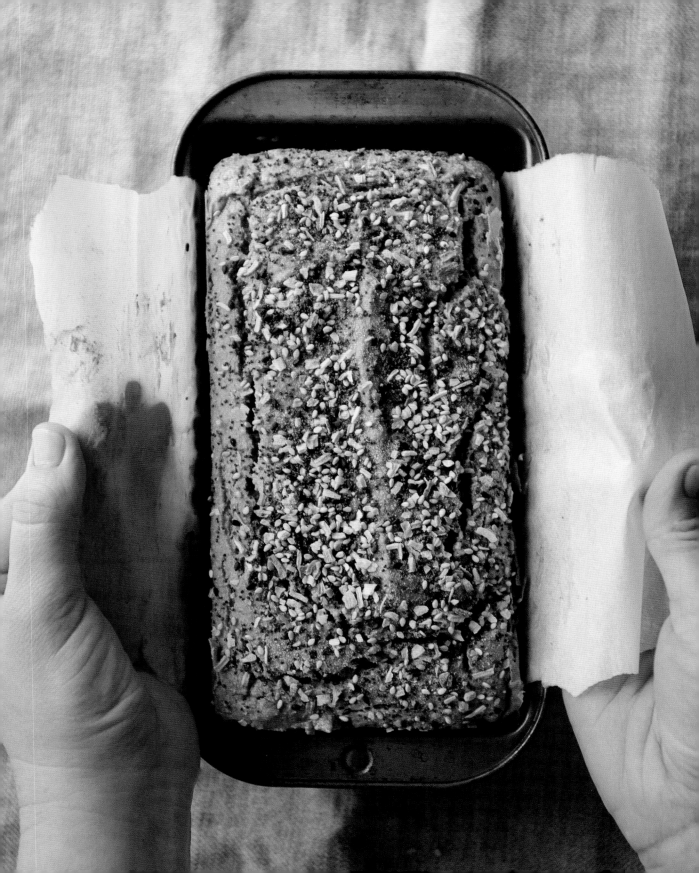

EVERYTHING BAGEL BREAD

Once you smell this bread baking in the oven, all bets are off! This recipe is the result of a strong craving Laurel had a year ago for an everything bagel with cream cheese—and when Laurel has a craving, that means she starts baking. Try this bread toasted with our herbed "cream cheese" that follows and you'll find your new favorite brunch snack. Now pass the lox!

MAKES ONE 9 × 5-INCH LOAF

½ cup plus 1 tablespoon almond flour

1 teaspoon baking soda

½ teaspoon Himalayan pink salt

1 cup tahini or cashew butter (page 38)

2 large eggs plus 2 large egg whites

1 tablespoon apple cider vinegar

1 teaspoon sesame seeds

1 teaspoon poppy seeds

1 teaspoon dehydrated garlic or garlic powder

1 teaspoon dehydrated onion or onion flakes

Herbed "Cream Cheese" (recipe follows), for serving

1. Preheat the oven to 350°F. Line a 9 × 5-inch loaf pan with parchment paper, letting the paper hang over the sides for easy removal, or grease the pan with coconut oil.

2. In a medium bowl, whisk together the flour, baking soda, and salt. In the bowl of a stand mixer fitted with the paddle attachment, beat the tahini, eggs, and egg whites until smooth. Slowly add 1 tablespoon water and the vinegar to the mixture on low speed. A little at a time, add the dry ingredients to the wet, beating on medium speed until well blended. Pour the batter into the prepared loaf pan.

3. In a small bowl, combine the sesame seeds, poppy seeds, garlic, and onion. Sprinkle the mixture evenly over the top of the batter. Bake for 20 to 30 minutes, until a toothpick inserted into the center comes out clean. Remove the bread from the pan, set on a rack, and allow to cool completely before slicing. Serve with herbed "cream cheese" for the full experience.

Herbed "Cream Cheese"

 MAKES 1 CUP

¾ cup whole raw cashews, soaked overnight in water

6 tablespoons coconut oil, solid

¼ cup fresh lemon juice

1 tablespoon tahini

1¼ teaspoons Himalayan pink salt

1 teaspoon chopped fresh chives

1 teaspoon chopped fresh mint leaves

1 teaspoon chopped fresh parsley

1 teaspoon chopped fresh dill

1 teaspoon freshly ground black pepper

1. Drain the cashews and place in a food processor with the coconut oil, lemon juice, tahini, and salt. Blend until creamy. If the mixture is too thick, add a little bit of water to loosen it up. Stir in the herbs and pepper by hand.

2. Place the mixture in a cheesecloth bag and lightly squeeze out any liquid. Transfer the "cream cheese" to a bowl or ramekin and refrigerate for at least 8 hours. Before serving, take out of the fridge for at least 2 hours to take the chill off, as coconut oil solidifies in the cold. Store in a sealed container in the fridge for up to a week.

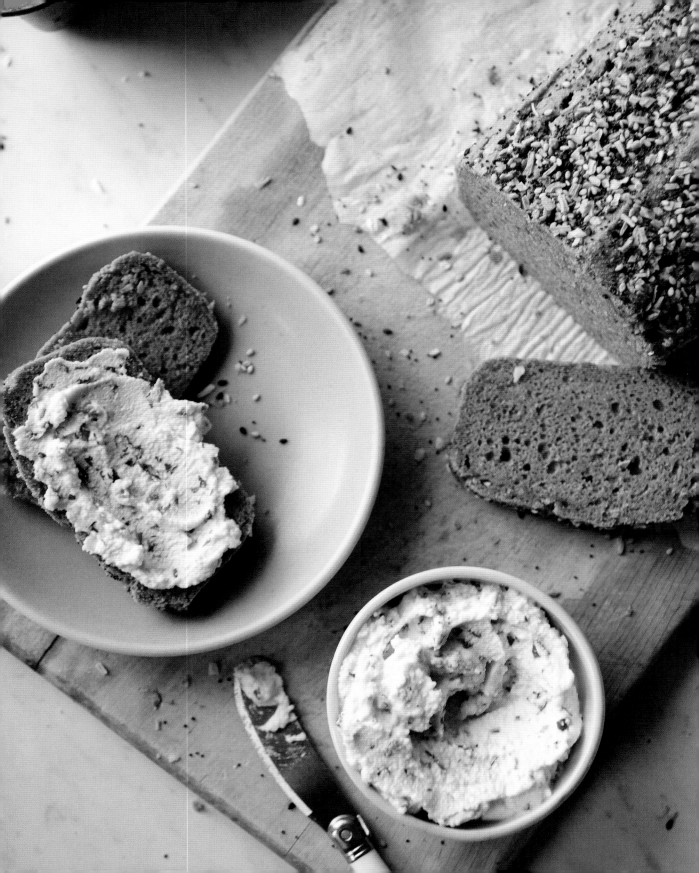

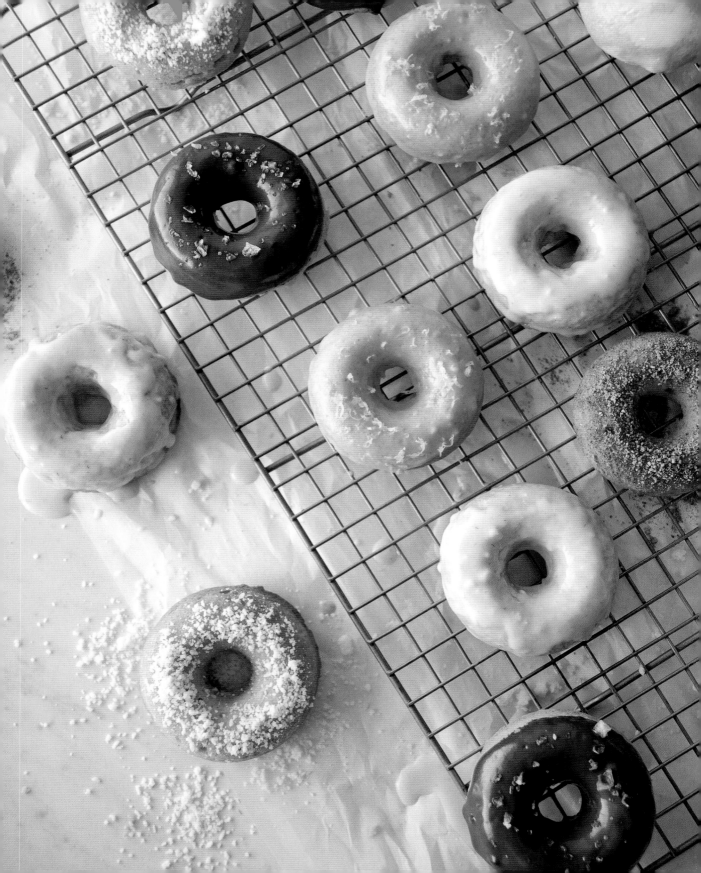

GLAZED DOUGHNUTS

If you're like us, doughnuts immediately take you back to your childhood. There was a mom in Claire's carpool who would take her on a surprise trip to the doughnut shop some mornings. These days were highlights of her childhood: standing behind the counter, trying to choose between all the mouthwatering options. Our recipe offers a variety of toppings, something we like at Sweet Laurel. These colorful, delicious doughnuts are a fun school-day surprise.

MAKES 12 LARGE DOUGHNUTS OR 18 SMALL DOUGHNUTS

Grass-fed ghee, for greasing the pan

Arrowroot powder, for dusting the pan

3 cups almond flour

½ teaspoon baking soda

¼ teaspoon Himalayan pink salt

¼ cup coconut oil, melted

½ cup coconut yogurt, store-bought or homemade (page 40)

⅓ cup maple syrup

1 teaspoon vanilla extract

2 teaspoons apple cider vinegar

4 large eggs, at room temperature, whites and yolks separated

Icing or glaze, for topping (recipes follow)

1. Preheat the oven to 350°F. Generously grease a doughnut pan with ghee and coat with arrowroot powder, shaking to discard any excess.

2. In a medium bowl, whisk together the flour, baking soda, and salt. In a large bowl, whisk together the coconut oil, coconut yogurt, maple syrup, vanilla, vinegar, and egg yolks. Gradually add the dry ingredients to the wet, stirring until just combined.

3. In another large bowl, beat the egg whites with a hand mixer until firm peaks form. Use a rubber spatula to gently fold the egg whites into the batter.

4. Pour the batter evenly into the doughnut molds, smoothing out the tops of each. Bake for 12 to 15 minutes, until light golden. Remove from the oven and let cool in the pan.

5. When the doughnuts have cooled completely, finish them with your favorite icing, glaze, or sugar.

Chocolate Glaze

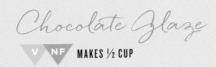 **MAKES ½ CUP**

5 ounces 100% cacao unsweetened baking chocolate, melted

1 tablespoon coconut oil, melted

2 tablespoons maple syrup

1. In a small bowl, combine all the ingredients and whisk until smooth.

2. Carefully dip each doughnut into the icing. Place on a rack to let the icing set, then serve.

Shredded Coconut "Powdered Sugar"

MAKES ¼ CUP

¼ cup unsweetened shredded coconut

2 teaspoons arrowroot powder

1. In a food processor, blend the coconut and arrowroot until a fine powder forms.

2. Sift the mixture over the doughnuts, generously dusting each, then serve.

Strawberry Icing

MAKES ¾ CUP

¼ cup coconut butter

2 teaspoons maple syrup or raw honey

1½ teaspoons fresh lemon juice

¼ teaspoon vanilla extract

¼ cup full-fat coconut milk

¼ cup strawberries, chopped

1. In a small saucepan, combine the coconut butter, maple syrup, ½ teaspoon of the lemon juice, the vanilla, and coconut milk over very low heat. Whisk until smooth. If the icing is too thick, add a little more coconut milk. If it's too runny, add more coconut butter.

2. In a small bowl, mash together the strawberries and the remaining 1 teaspoon fresh lemon juice with the back of a fork. Push the strawberries through a strainer into the icing, then stir to combine.

3. Carefully dip each doughnut into the icing. Place on a rack to let the icing set, then serve.

Turmeric Lemon Glaze

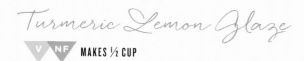 **MAKES ½ CUP**

¼ cup coconut butter

2 teaspoons maple syrup or raw honey

2 teaspoons fresh lemon juice

¼ teaspoon vanilla extract

¼ cup full-fat coconut milk

½ teaspoon turmeric

½ teaspoon grated lemon zest, for garnish

1. In a small saucepan, combine the coconut butter, maple syrup, lemon juice, vanilla, coconut milk, and turmeric over very low heat. Whisk until smooth. If the icing is too thick, add a little more coconut milk. If it's too runny, add more coconut butter.

2. Carefully dip each doughnut into the icing. Place on a rack and sprinkle the lemon zest over the doughnuts. Let the icing set, then serve.

Coconut Butter Icing

MAKES ½ CUP

¼ cup coconut butter

2 teaspoons maple syrup or raw honey

½ teaspoon fresh lemon juice

¼ teaspoon vanilla extract

¼ cup full-fat coconut milk

1. In a small saucepan, combine all the ingredients over very low heat. Whisk until smooth. If the icing is too thick, add a little more coconut milk. If it's too runny, add more coconut butter.

2. Carefully dip each doughnut into the icing. Place on a rack to let the icing set, then serve.

—Notes—

If they're not freshly baked, briefly warm the doughnuts in the oven before topping with the date sugar mixture.

Date sugar is simply dehydrated dates broken down, and when used as garnish, coconut sugar can be used instead, though the caramel flavor is not as pronounced.

Cinnamon Date Sugar

MAKES ½ CUP

½ cup date sugar

½ teaspoon ground cinnamon

1. Whisk together the date sugar and cinnamon, then spread out on a baking sheet.

2. Roll the warm doughnuts through the mixture, pressing lightly to help the sugar adhere. Place on a rack to cool, then serve.

STRAWBERRY-STUFFED FRENCH TOAST

A lazy Sunday morning just wouldn't be complete without the scent of French toast sizzling in the pan waking you up. We take our rendition a step further with the delightful addition of jam between layers of bread. It's sweet, bright, crisp, and satisfying all in one bite. This recipe is perfect with bread that's a day or two old—it actually soaks the batter up better than if it were fresh!

SERVES 4

Eight ½-inch slices sandwich bread, store-bought or homemade (page 53)

1 cup berry jam, store-bought or homemade (page 208)

4 large eggs

¼ cup full-fat coconut milk

1½ teaspoons ground cinnamon

¼ cup maple syrup

Pinch of Himalayan pink salt

1 to 2 tablespoons coconut oil

Coconut Whipped Cream (page 30), sliced strawberries, and maple syrup, for serving

1. Sandwich 2 slices of bread with however much jam you please. Repeat with the remaining bread and jam.

2. In a large, shallow bowl, whisk together the eggs, coconut milk, cinnamon, maple syrup, and salt. Dunk the sandwiches into the egg mixture one at a time, soaking for 10 seconds on each side.

3. In a large skillet over medium heat, melt enough coconut oil to cover the bottom of the pan. Put as many sandwiches as will fit in the pan and cook for about 5 minutes on each side, until crisped and golden brown. Repeat with the remaining sandwiches, adding more oil if necessary.

4. Serve the French toast hot with a generous helping of coconut whipped cream, some sliced strawberries, and a drizzle of maple syrup on top.

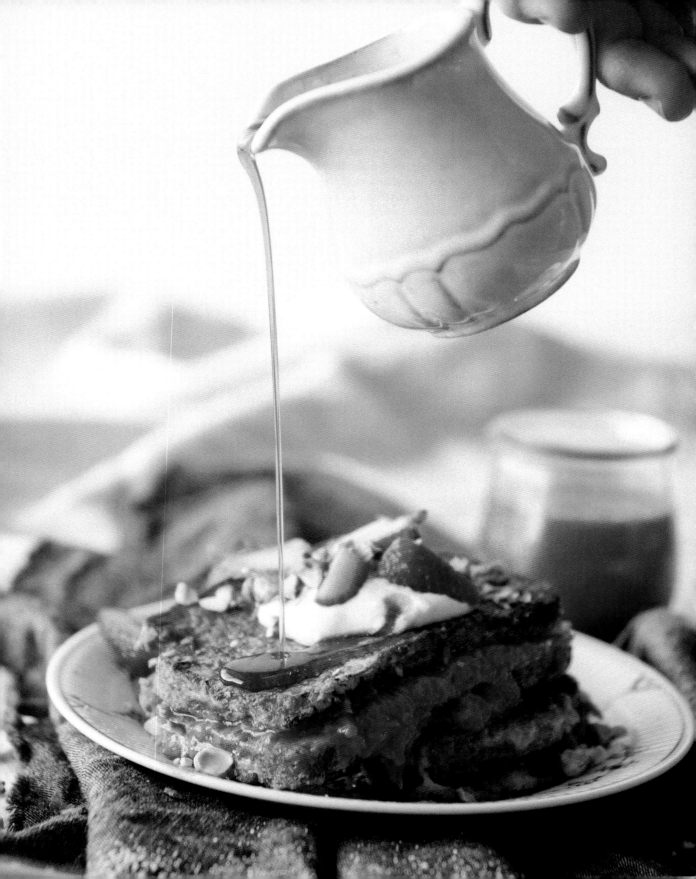

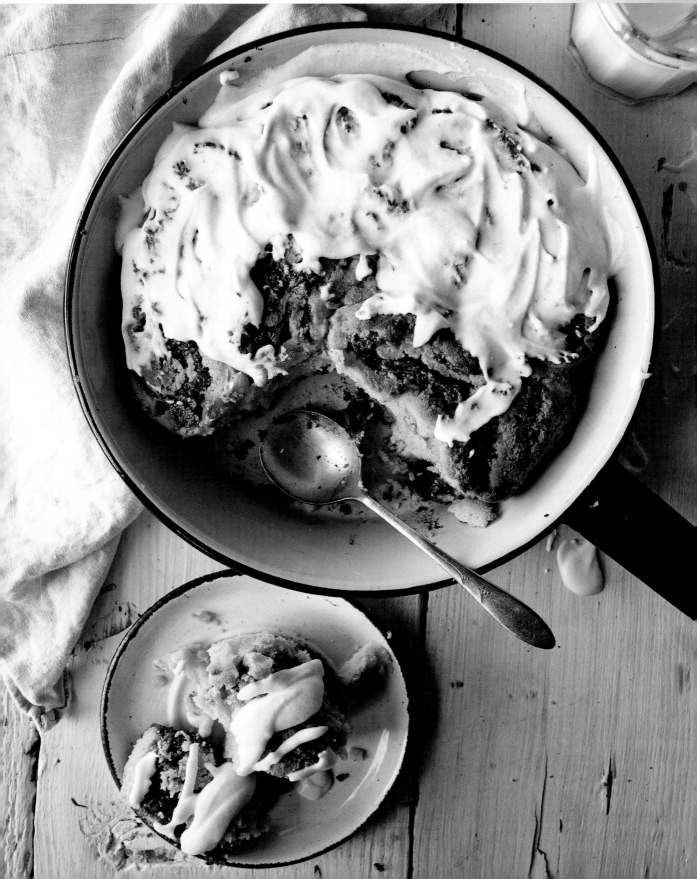

FOR THE FILLING

1½ cups date paste, store-bought or homemade (page 42)

⅔ cup maple syrup, plus more as needed

1½ tablespoons ground cinnamon

1 tablespoon vanilla extract

Coconut oil, for greasing the parchment and pan

Coconut Cream Cheese Glaze (page 218)

7. **MAKE THE FILLING:** Combine the date paste, maple syrup, cinnamon, and vanilla in a food processor and pulse until smooth and thin enough to spread. If you need it thinner, just add a little more maple syrup, pulsing again.

8. Remove the dough from the refrigerator. Let the dough rest while you preheat the oven to 350°F. Roll out a large piece of parchment paper, about 2 feet long, and grease well with coconut oil. Press the dough onto the parchment paper, cover with another piece of parchment, and roll it about ⅓ inch thick. Remove the top piece of parchment and spoon on the date filling, gently smoothing it evenly, but leaving a ¼-inch border all around. Don't press too hard, as the dough will be quite soft.

9. **CREATE THE ROLLS:** Lift the long edge of the parchment, and gently fold the dough over, covering the first inch of the date filling. Then, using the parchment to help you, continue rolling the dough over itself until you've created a parchment-covered log. Refrigerate the log for about an hour, to set the dough and make it easier to slice.

10. Grease a large ovenproof skillet with coconut oil. Take out the log and gently unwrap it. The dough will want to stick to the parchment, so use a butter knife to separate it from the paper. With a greased knife, cut the log into 1½-inch slices; you should end up with 15 to 17 rolls. Place the rolls in the skillet, side by side. The skillet should look filled but with some gaps, not crammed with dough.

11. Bake the rolls for 20 to 30 minutes, until golden brown and firm to the touch. If you do the toothpick test, be sure to poke the toothpick just in the roll portion, not the date filling. The filling will leave the toothpick gooey, and you won't get an accurate read on the rolls' doneness.

12. Remove the rolls from the oven and coat with the coconut cream cheese glaze in the pan. Serve warm. If making the rolls for later, don't glaze them; cover and refrigerate for up to 3 days. Reheat and glaze the rolls just before serving.

Notes

You can press the pause button and make these delicious rolls ahead of time. The filling and the glaze can be prepped beforehand as well.

Expect to see the dough puff up a bit, about 50 percent at a time, rather than very dramatically. This is due to the heaviness of the almond flour and the small amount of maple syrup.

NUT-MILK PORRIDGE

In recent years, savory porridge has become a huge trend, but porridge is almost never grain- or gluten-free. To get that same comforting, creamy texture, we cook our favorite nuts with some chia seeds and flaxseed meal to help bind everything together. This is a simple recipe that works beautifully with any ingredient combination: poached eggs and market vegetables? Done! Want to sweeten it up with fresh fruit and raw honey? Go for it. This is a recipe to play with.

SERVES 4

1 cup cashews

1 cup pecans

1½ cups almond milk

1 tablespoon chia seeds

1 tablespoon flaxseed meal

2 tablespoons unsweetened shredded coconut

⅛ teaspoon Himalayan pink salt

Savory Granola (recipe follows) and fresh fruit, for garnish

1. Coarsely grind the cashews and pecans in a food processor. Be sure to gently pulse the nuts, lest they turn into nut butter.

2. Pour the almond milk into a medium saucepan over medium heat and bring to a simmer. Add the chia seeds, flax, coconut, and salt, as well as the ground nut mixture, and stir to combine. Simmer for 10 minutes, or until the nuts are softened and the chia seeds slightly puffed up.

3. Serve the porridge warm, with plenty of granola on top.

Savory Granola

MAKES 3½ CUPS

This recipe is meant to be a canvas, so serve with roasted sweet potatoes from last night's dinner or chunks of avocado and hot sauce. Or, if you're in a sweet mood, just add a little maple syrup to the granola for a more classic version.

1 cup almonds

1 cup walnuts

1 cup pecans

½ teaspoon Himalayan pink salt

½ cup unsweetened shredded coconut

¼ cup sesame seeds

¼ cup coconut oil, melted

2 large egg whites

1 tablespoon coconut aminos (see page 249)

1. Preheat the oven to 350°F. Line a baking sheet with parchment paper.

2. Coarsely grind the almonds, walnuts, and pecans together in a food processor. Place the ground nuts in a medium bowl and stir in the salt, coconut, sesame seeds, and coconut oil.

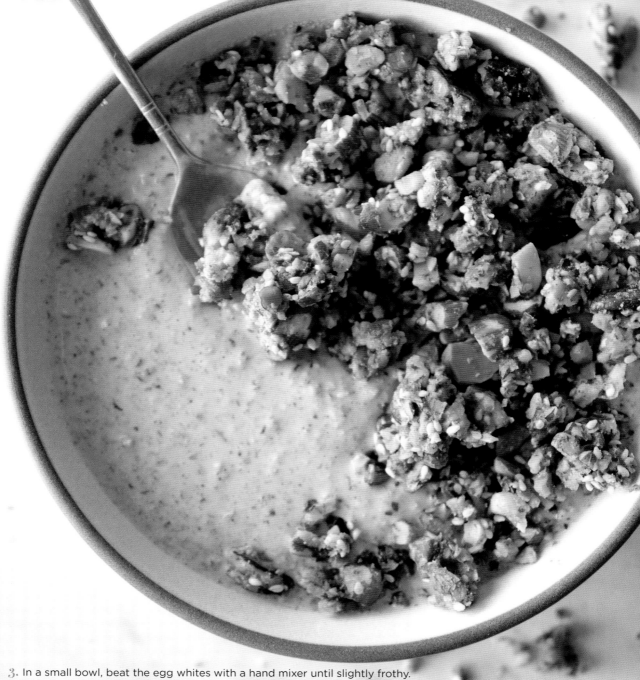

3. In a small bowl, beat the egg whites with a hand mixer until slightly frothy. Pour the egg whites into the nut mixture, add the coconut aminos, and stir.

4. Pour the granola onto the prepared pan and use a spatula to spread it out to cover the entire surface. Bake for about 15 to 20 minutes, until golden brown, fragrant, and crunchy. Break into pieces. Let the granola cool and harden for about 20 minutes. Store in an airtight container for up to 3 days.

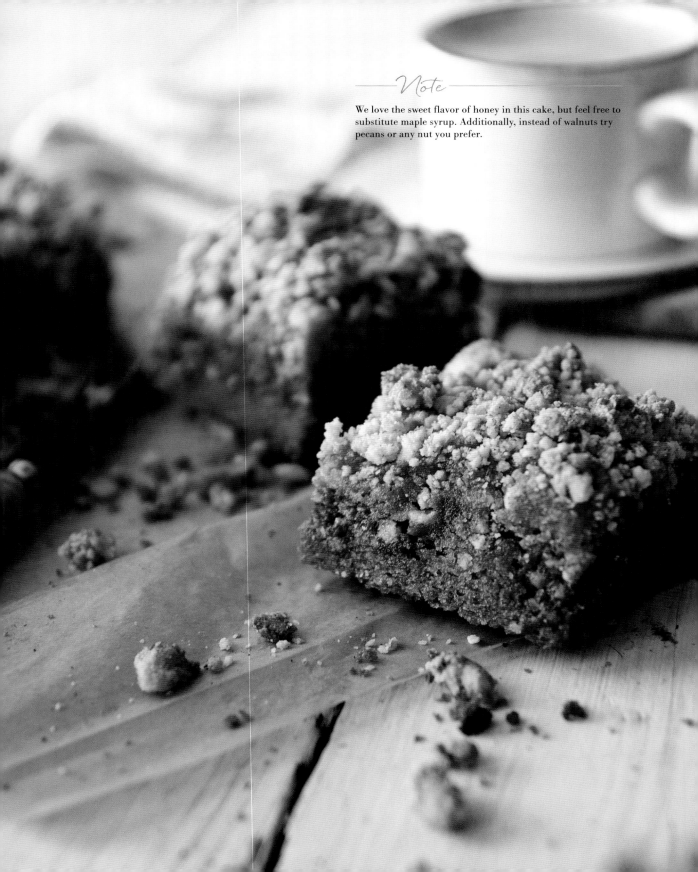

We love the sweet flavor of honey in this cake, but feel free to substitute maple syrup. Additionally, instead of walnuts try pecans or any nut you prefer.

HONEY-WALNUT COFFEE CAKE

We are the people who eat the tops of muffins first and who pick the streusel off a cake, because that sweet, caramelized crunch is our favorite texture. And a good coffee cake requires a thick layer of streusel on top. The crunch is an important contrast to the moist cake and sticky, sweet cinnamon filling. This delicious cake hits all of our marks and is the perfect complement to a simple cup of coffee.

MAKES ONE 8-INCH CAKE

FOR THE STREUSEL

¾ cup almond flour

¾ cup chopped walnuts

3 tablespoons coconut oil, melted

3 tablespoons maple syrup

1 teaspoon ground cinnamon

¼ teaspoon Himalayan pink salt

FOR THE CAKE

⅓ cup coconut oil, melted

⅔ cup honey

4 large eggs

2 teaspoons vanilla extract

3 cups almond flour

1 teaspoon baking soda

½ teaspoon Himalayan pink salt

FOR THE FILLING

1 cup chopped walnuts

¼ cup coconut oil, melted

½ cup honey

2 tablespoons ground cinnamon

Pinch of Himalayan pink salt

1. Preheat the oven to 350°F. Line a baking sheet with parchment paper for the streusel. Line an 8 × 8-inch pan with parchment paper, letting the paper hang over the sides for easy removal.

2. **MAKE THE STREUSEL:** In a small bowl, whisk together the flour, walnuts, coconut oil, maple syrup, cinnamon, and salt until the mixture comes together. Crumble onto the baking sheet and bake for 10 minutes or until the streusel begins to crisp up. Remove and set aside, but keep the oven on at 350°F.

3. **MAKE THE CAKE:** In a large bowl, whisk together the coconut oil, honey, eggs, and vanilla until smooth. In a medium bowl, whisk together the flour, baking soda, and salt. A little at a time, add the dry ingredients to the wet, stirring to combine. Pour half of the batter into the prepared pan, smoothing it with a spatula.

4. **MAKE THE FILLING:** In a medium bowl, stir together the walnuts, coconut oil, honey, cinnamon, and salt and spoon over the batter, coating the surface as best you can. Pour on the second half of the batter, and then scatter the streusel over the top.

5. Bake for 25 minutes, then cover with foil and continue baking for another 20 minutes, or until the streusel is golden brown and the cake is puffed and firm. The toothpick test won't give you an accurate read on doneness as it will come out gooey because of the filling. Once the cake is cooled in the pan, lift it out with the parchment paper and slice into squares. To save for later, wrap in plastic and keep at room temperature for up to 3 days, but it's best the same day it's baked.

SESAME CRACKERS

These are our absolute favorite crackers—we're addicted to the sesame flavor in these nutty little bites. Topped with avocado, they make a delicious snack, or served with our nut-milk cheese, they make for a sophisticated cheese board. We also find ourselves munching on these after yoga for a little refueling.

MAKES 3 DOZEN THICK CRACKERS OR 6 DOZEN THIN CRACKERS

2½ cups almond flour

1 teaspoon Himalayan pink salt

¾ cup brown sesame seeds

¼ cup black sesame seeds

1 tablespoon flaxseeds

2 tablespoons coconut oil, melted

2 large eggs

Nut-Milk Cheese (recipe follows), for serving

1. Preheat the oven to 350°F.

2. In a medium bowl, whisk together the flour, salt, and seeds. In a separate medium bowl, combine the coconut oil and eggs. A little at a time, add the dry ingredients to the wet, stirring until a dough comes together.

3. Place the dough between two large pieces of parchment paper. For thick crackers, roll the dough about ¼ inch thick; for thin crackers, 1/16 inch thick. Transfer the dough and bottom layer of parchment to a baking sheet. Use a paring knife to cut the dough into squares. Don't worry about separating them, you can easily break them apart after baking. Bake thick crackers for 14 to 15 minutes and thin for 12 to 13 minutes, or until golden brown and crisp. Let the crackers cool completely before serving with the "cheese."

Nut-Milk Cheese

MAKES 1 CUP

¾ cup raw cashews, soaked overnight in water

6 tablespoons coconut oil, solid

1 tablespoon fresh lemon juice

1 tablespoon tahini

1¼ teaspoons Himalayan pink salt

1. Drain the cashews and place in a food processor with the coconut oil, lemon juice, tahini, and salt. Blend until creamy. If the mixture is too thick, add a little bit of water to loosen it up.

2. Place the mixture in a cheesecloth or nut-milk bag and lightly squeeze out any liquid. Transfer the cheese to a small bowl and refrigerate until ready to serve. Before serving, take out of the fridge for at least 2 hours to take the chill off, as coconut oil solidifies in the cold. Store in a sealed container in the fridge for up to a week.

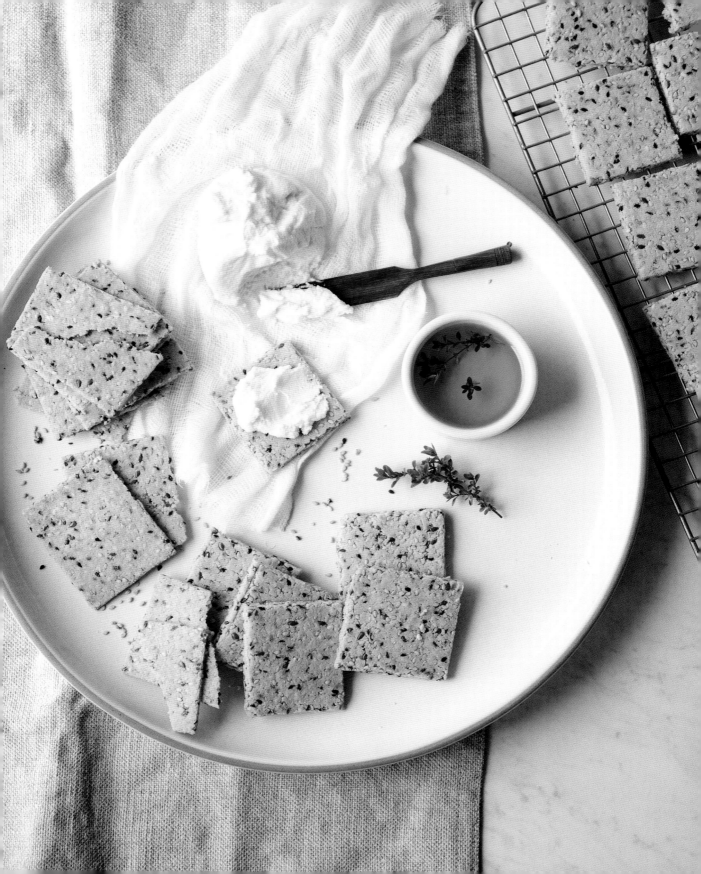

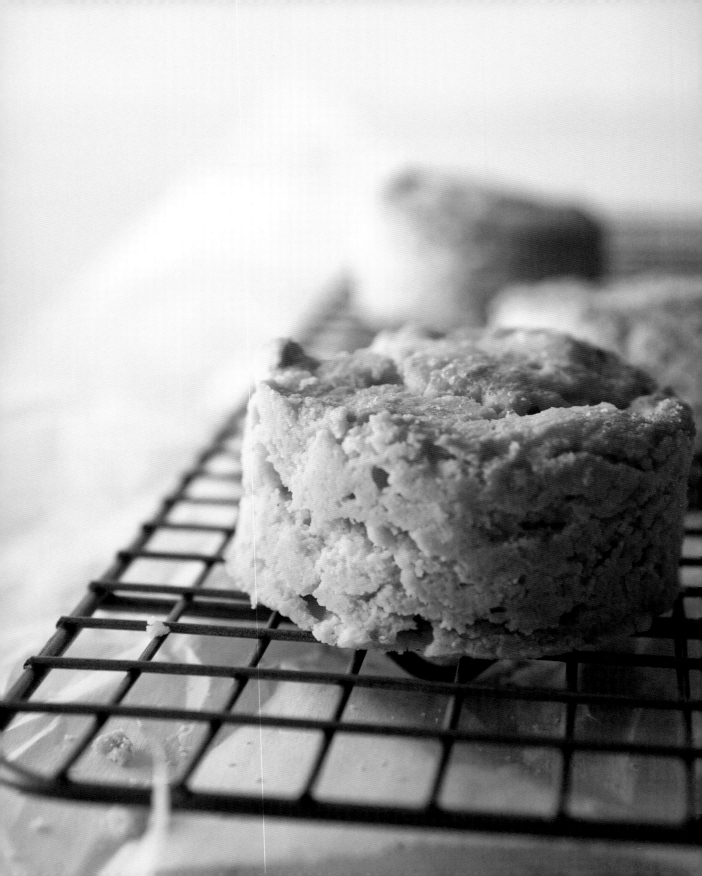

SOUTHERN BISCUITS

Buttery, flaky biscuits are a challenge in grain-free baking, but we cracked the code. Funny enough, we took our favorite classic biscuit recipe and simply swapped in Sweet Laurel–approved ingredients, which usually doesn't work. Guess this just proves that biscuits are a little bit magical!

MAKES EIGHT 3-INCH BISCUITS

2 tablespoons coconut butter, cubed

2 tablespoons coconut oil, solid

2½ cups almond flour

1 tablespoon baking powder

½ teaspoon Himalayan pink salt

¾ cup coconut yogurt, store-bought or homemade (page 40)

1 large egg, beaten

1. Preheat the oven to 350°F. Line a baking sheet with parchment paper.

2. Combine the coconut butter and coconut oil in a small bowl and chill in the freezer for about 5 minutes.

3. In a medium bowl, whisk together the flour, baking powder, and salt. Add the chilled coconut butter and coconut oil and cut in using a pastry blender, until a meal forms. It will look like wet sand, and the fats should be pea sized. Stir in the coconut yogurt. Loosely form the dough into a ball and place on a sheet of parchment paper.

4. Cover the dough with a second sheet of parchment paper and press into a ¾-inch-thick rectangle. Fold the dough over onto itself in three sections, like you would a letter. Again pat down the dough until it's ¾ inch thick, and repeat this entire process two more times. This creates the fluffy layers that will puff and add lift as the biscuits bake.

5. Press out the folded dough so it's 1 inch thick, and cut out biscuits with a 3-inch round cookie cutter or the rim of a juice glass. Place the rounds on the prepared baking sheet.

6. Using a pastry brush, lightly coat the top of each biscuit with the beaten egg. Bake for about 15 minutes, or until puffed up and golden. Allow to cool or serve warm.

MIXED BERRY BREAKFAST TARTS

Breakfast cake is a tradition at Sweet Laurel, so breakfast pie seemed like a step in the right direction. Because our ingredients are wholesome and filling, there aren't any sugary, empty calories—our breakfast tarts are actually a delicious, sweet option to pair with your morning cup of coffee. The crust is flaky and tender, the filling is tart and fresh, and a pretty pink glaze finishes everything perfectly.

MAKES 4 TARTS

FOR THE CRUST

2½ cups almond flour

1 cup arrowroot powder

Pinch of Himalayan pink salt

¼ cup coconut oil, solid

¼ cup maple syrup

1 large egg

FOR THE FILLING

1½ cups fresh or frozen mixed berries

¼ cup maple syrup

Juice of ½ lemon

1 teaspoon arrowroot powder

1 large egg, beaten with a teaspoon of water, for egg wash

Strawberry Icing (page 66), for garnish

Paleo Sprinkles (page 224), for garnish

1. **MAKE THE CRUST:** In a medium bowl, whisk together the flour, arrowroot powder, and salt. Cut the coconut oil into the dry ingredients with a pastry blender or your fingertips until a dough comes together. It will look like wet sand, and the fats should be pea sized. Add the maple syrup and egg, and stir into a dough. Gently shape the dough into a ball, cover with plastic wrap, press into a disk, and chill in the fridge for about 2 hours.

2. Preheat the oven to 350°F. Line a baking sheet with parchment paper.

3. Place the dough between two pieces of parchment paper and roll it about ⅛ inch thick. Remove the top piece of parchment and, using a paring knife, cut the dough into 8 matching rectangles, about 4 × 5 inches. Place the dough on the prepared baking sheet and chill in the refrigerator while you prepare the filling.

4. **MAKE THE FILLING:** In a medium saucepan over medium heat, combine the berries, maple syrup, and lemon juice. Cook for about 10 minutes, until the mixture begins to boil, then remove from the heat and stir in the arrowroot powder. Let the mixture cool to room temperature, about 30 minutes.

5. Place 2 tablespoons of the berry mixture in the center of 4 of the dough rectangles. Place another rectangle on top of each and seal together by crimping the edges with fork tines. Use a fork to prick air vents in the top of the dough.

6. Brush the egg wash lightly over each pastry and bake for 20 to 30 minutes, until golden brown and any berry liquid dripping out appears thick. Glaze with strawberry icing and decorate with sprinkles.

Note

Inspired by toaster pastries, these can be made ahead of time. Refrigerate before you add the icing and sprinkles for up to 2 days. Rewarm before serving, and finish with the icing and sprinkles.

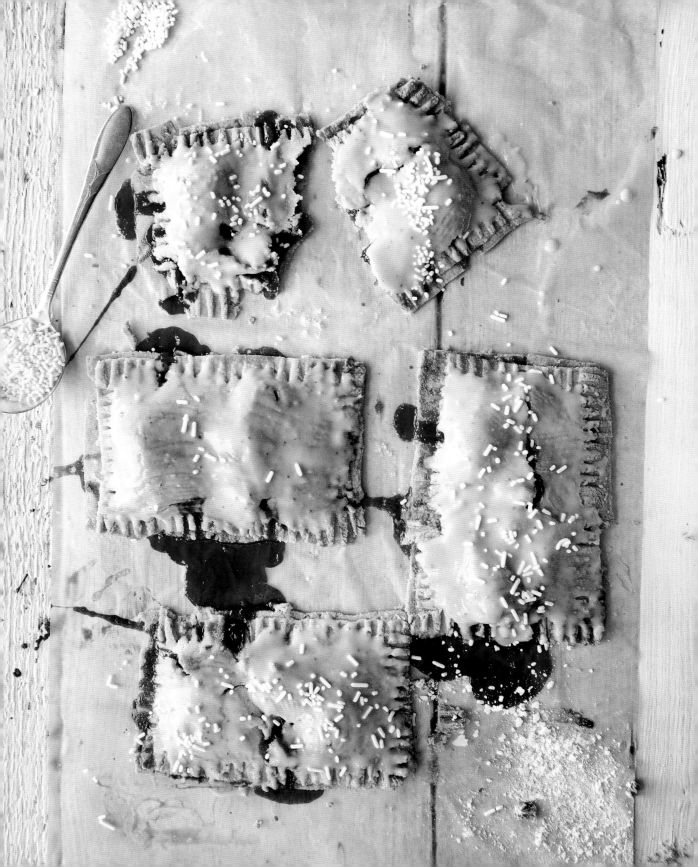

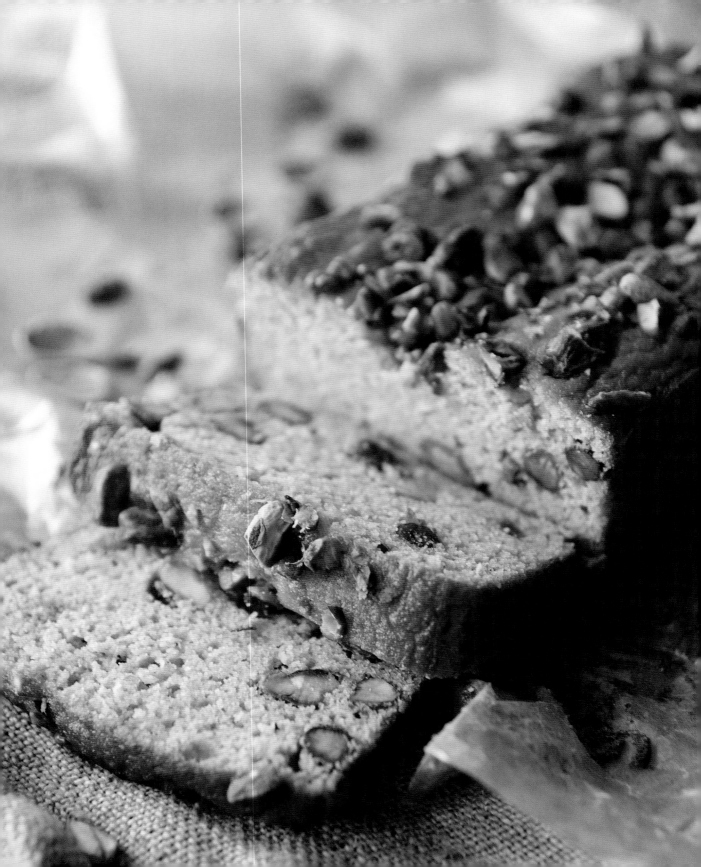

ORANGE PISTACHIO LOAF

Laurel's orange loaf was the third recipe to appear in the Sweet Laurel recipe catalog. (First was The Chocolate Cake That Changed Everything, page 167, and second was the Blueberry Streusel Muffins, page 51.) We've baked it with different nuts, dried fruit, even chocolate chips, but we especially love it studded with pistachios. We've been known to accidentally eat an entire mini loaf by ourselves for breakfast, and if you somehow manage to have leftovers, you'll find this loaf is delicious toasted and drizzled with honey the next day.

MAKES FIVE 3 × 5-INCH MINI LOAVES OR ONE 9 × 5-INCH LOAF

¾ cup coconut flour

1 teaspoon baking soda

½ teaspoon Himalayan pink salt

¼ cup coconut oil, melted

6 large eggs

½ cup orange juice (from about 2 oranges)

Grated zest of 1 orange

½ cup pure maple syrup

1 teaspoon vanilla extract

½ cup whole raw pistachios

¼ cup chopped raw pistachios

1. Preheat the oven to 350°F. Line either 5 mini loaf pans or one 9 × 5-inch loaf pan with parchment paper, letting the paper hang over the sides for easy removal, or grease the pans with coconut oil.

2. In a large bowl, whisk together the flour, baking soda, and salt. In a separate large bowl, whisk the coconut oil, eggs, orange juice and zest, maple syrup, and vanilla. A little at a time, add the dry ingredients to the wet, stirring until a batter forms. Fold in the whole pistachios.

3. Pour the batter into the prepared pans and sprinkle the chopped pistachios on top. Bake for 15 to 20 minutes for the mini loaves and 30 to 40 minutes for a large loaf, until a toothpick inserted into the center comes out clean. Remove the bread from the pans, set on a rack, and let cool to room temperature before serving.

STONEFRUIT CLAFOUTIS

A summertime farmer's market makes us immediately think of this simple French breakfast sweet. If you haven't had it before, imagine a cross between a baked pancake and a flan, studded with fresh fruit. The classic version of clafoutis is made with ripe black cherries, pits included, which add a subtle almond flavor to the light, eggy batter. Our version is made with almond flour and seasonal fruit, so the flavors of sweet, bright fresh fruit and almond are still there.

MAKES ONE 9-INCH PAN

3 tablespoons coconut oil, melted, plus more for greasing the pan

1 cup full-fat coconut milk

¼ cup maple syrup

2 teaspoons vanilla extract

¼ teaspoon apple cider vinegar

1¼ cups almond flour

1 teaspoon baking powder

¼ teaspoon Himalayan pink salt

4 large eggs

2 cups sliced fresh fruit (we used stone fruit and figs)

Shredded Coconut "Powdered Sugar" (page 66), for garnish

1. Preheat the oven to 350°F. Grease a 9-inch ovenproof skillet with coconut oil.

2. Combine the coconut oil, coconut milk, maple syrup, vanilla, vinegar, flour, baking powder, salt, and eggs in a blender and pulse until a smooth batter forms.

3. Scatter the fruit across the skillet. Pour the batter over it. Bake for 50 to 55 minutes, until the clafoutis is puffed and golden brown.

4. Serve the clafoutis hot with more fresh fruit and lots of coconut powdered sugar.

Note

This recipe can be made with any peak-of-season fruit, but we especially love it with cherries, plums, or figs.

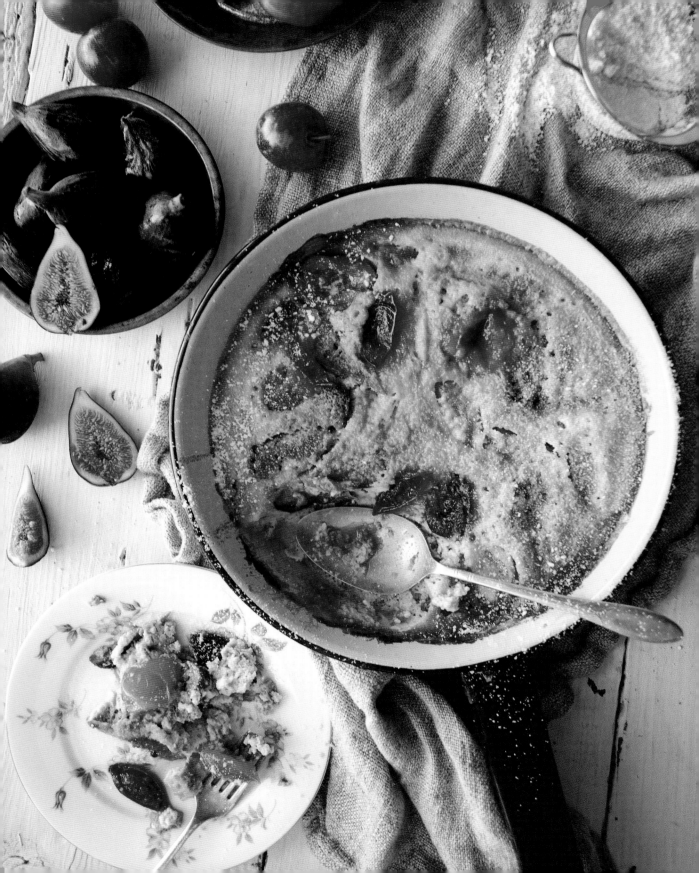

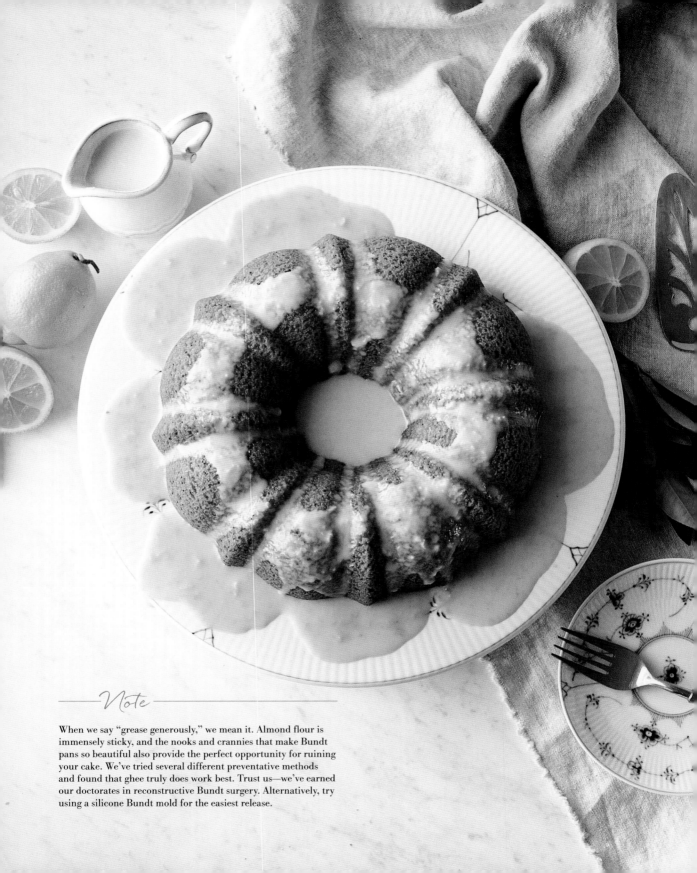

— *Note* —

When we say "grease generously," we mean it. Almond flour is immensely sticky, and the nooks and crannies that make Bundt pans so beautiful also provide the perfect opportunity for ruining your cake. We've tried several different preventative methods and found that ghee truly does work best. Trust us—we've earned our doctorates in reconstructive Bundt surgery. Alternatively, try using a silicone Bundt mold for the easiest release.

LEMON POPPYSEED BUNDT

It's a Bundt! That's Laurel's favorite line from *My Big Fat Greek Wedding*, and this is one of Claire's favorite recipes in the book, so get ready for something delicious. If you have friends or family who side-eye grain-free baked goods, this is the recipe to make for them—we doubt they'll miss anything. Lemon-scented with nutty notes of poppyseed, this cake is the perfect complement to a cup of coffee and friends on a Sunday afternoon.

MAKES ONE 9-INCH BUNDT CAKE

Grass-fed ghee or coconut oil, for greasing the pan

Arrowroot powder, for dusting the pan

4 cups almond flour

½ teaspoon Himalayan pink salt

1 teaspoon baking soda

3 large eggs

¾ cup full-fat coconut milk

1 cup maple syrup

2 tablespoons grated lemon zest

¼ cup fresh lemon juice

2 tablespoons poppy seeds

Coconut Butter Glaze (recipe follows)

1. Preheat the oven to 350°F. Generously grease a 9-inch Bundt pan with ghee and coat with arrowroot powder, shaking to discard any excess.

2. In a medium bowl, whisk the flour, salt, and baking soda. In a large bowl, whisk together the eggs, coconut milk, maple syrup, lemon zest, and lemon juice until combined. A little at a time, add the dry ingredients to the wet, stirring well until a batter forms; then stir in the poppy seeds.

3. Pour the batter into the greased pan and bake for 40 to 50 minutes, or until golden brown and a toothpick inserted into the center comes out clean. Allow the cake to cool in the pan for about an hour. Invert the bundt onto a plate to release the cake. Drizzle the glaze over the cooled cake, then cut and serve.

Coconut Butter Glaze

V NF MAKES ½ CUP

¼ cup coconut butter

2 teaspoons maple syrup or raw honey

½ teaspoon fresh lemon juice

¼ teaspoon vanilla extract

¼ cup full-fat coconut milk or almond milk

Combine all the ingredients in a small saucepan over low heat, stirring for 10 minutes, or until blended together. If you want thinner icing, add more coconut milk. For a thicker glaze, add more coconut butter. Allow the glaze to cool completely before drizzling over the cake.

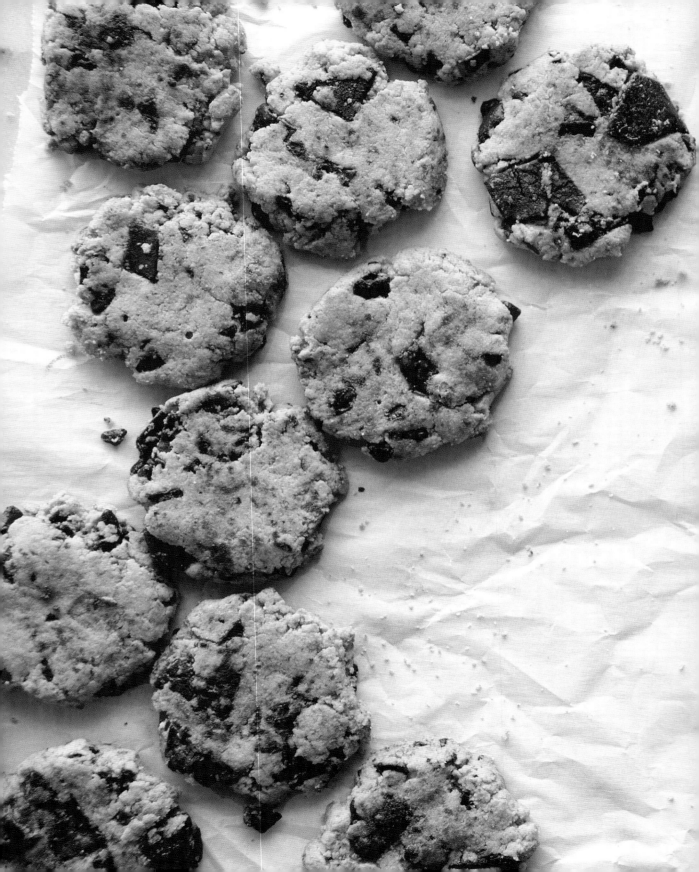

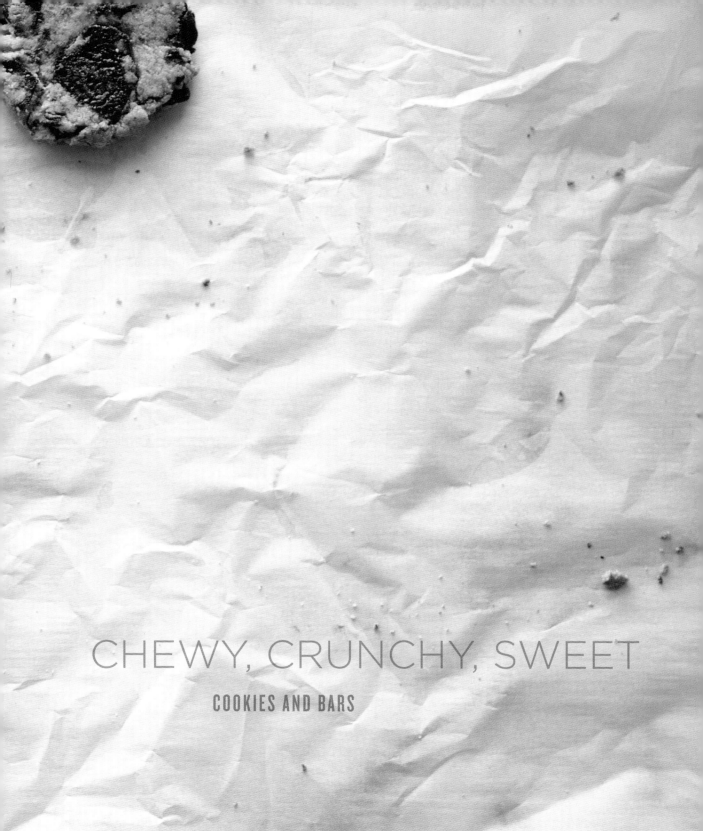

CHEWY, CRUNCHY, SWEET

COOKIES AND BARS

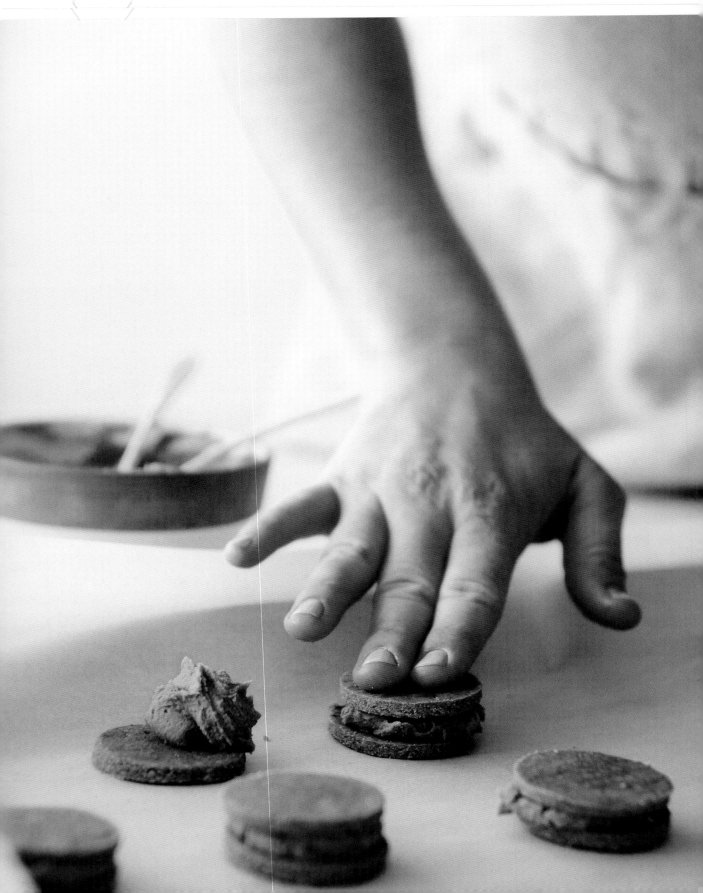

MATCHA SANDWICH COOKIES

When we first fell in love with matcha, we just had to find a way to incorporate the antioxidant-rich superfood into our baked goods. These little sandwich cookies are the perfect treat with a hot cup of tea—make it a hot cup of matcha for an extra boost! For the best color and flavor, use fresh, bright green matcha.

MAKES 1 DOZEN SANDWICH COOKIES

FOR THE COOKIES

2 cups almond flour

1/8 teaspoon Himalayan pink salt

1/4 cup coconut oil, melted

1/4 cup maple syrup

1 teaspoon matcha powder

FOR THE FILLING

1/4 cup coconut butter

2 teaspoons maple syrup or raw honey

1/2 teaspoon fresh lemon juice

1/4 teaspoon vanilla extract

1/4 cup full-fat coconut milk

1 teaspoon matcha powder

1. Preheat the oven to 350°F. Line a baking sheet with parchment paper.

2. **MAKE THE COOKIES:** In a large bowl, whisk together the flour and salt. In a medium bowl, combine the coconut oil and maple syrup. A little at a time, add the dry ingredients to the wet, stirring until a dough comes together. Gradually stir in the matcha, being sure to break up any lumps.

3. Place the dough between two pieces of parchment paper and roll it about 1/8 inch thick. Remove the top piece of paper and, using a 1 1/2-inch or 2-inch round cookie cutter, cut the dough into circles and place on the prepared baking sheet. Bake for 7 to 9 minutes, until the edges begin turning golden brown. Transfer the cookies to a rack to cool completely while you prepare the filling.

4. **MAKE THE FILLING:** In a small saucepan, combine the coconut butter, maple syrup, lemon juice, vanilla, and coconut milk. Cook over very low heat, stirring occasionally, until the mixture is smooth and thick. Remove the pan from the heat and whisk in the matcha. Let the filling cool to room temperature.

5. Gently spread 1 to 2 teaspoons of filling onto a cooled matcha cookie, then top with another cookie. Repeat with the remaining cookies and serve. Store in a sealed container at room temperature for up to 5 days, or in the freezer indefinitely.

LAVENDER SANDWICH COOKIES

These are the most ladylike cookies. We first made them for a tea party with our girlfriends, and they were gone in minutes. They are soft and chewy, with a slight hint of delicate lavender in every bite. Be sure to use food-grade lavender oil, as not all essential oils are meant for ingestion. (And no one likes a soapy-tasting cookie!) If you can't find lavender oil, use food-grade dried lavender. You'll see little flecks of the flowers in the dough, and they will still have that delicate, soothing floral flavor. These are especially good with a cup of Earl Grey tea.

MAKES 1 DOZEN SANDWICH COOKIES

FOR THE COOKIES

2½ cups almond flour

¼ teaspoon Himalayan pink salt

1 tablespoon ground culinary lavender

¼ cup coconut oil, melted

¼ cup maple syrup

½ teaspoon vanilla extract

FOR THE FILLING

1 drop culinary lavender oil, or 1 teaspoon ground culinary lavender

¼ cup coconut butter

2 teaspoons maple syrup or raw honey

½ teaspoon fresh lemon juice

¼ teaspoon vanilla extract

¼ cup full-fat coconut milk

1. Preheat the oven to 350°F. Line a baking sheet with parchment paper.

2. **MAKE THE COOKIES:** In a medium bowl, whisk together the flour, salt, and lavender. In a medium bowl, combine the coconut oil, maple syrup, and vanilla. A little at a time, add the dry ingredients to the wet, stirring until a dough comes together.

3. Place the dough between two pieces of parchment paper and roll it about ⅛ inch thick. Remove the top piece of paper and, using a 1½-inch round cookie cutter, cut the dough into circles and place on the prepared baking sheet. Bake for 7 to 9 minutes, until the edges begin turning golden brown. Transfer the cookies to a rack to cool completely while you make the filling.

4. **MAKE THE FILLING:** In a small saucepan, combine the lavender oil, coconut butter, maple syrup, lemon juice, vanilla, and coconut milk. Cook over very low heat, stirring occasionally, until smooth, about 5 to 7 minutes. Remove the pan from the heat and let the filling cool to room temperature.

5. Gently spread 1 to 2 teaspoons of filling onto a cooled lavender cookie, then top with another cookie. Repeat with the remaining cookies and serve. Store in a sealed container at room temperature for up to 5 days, or in the freezer indefinitely.

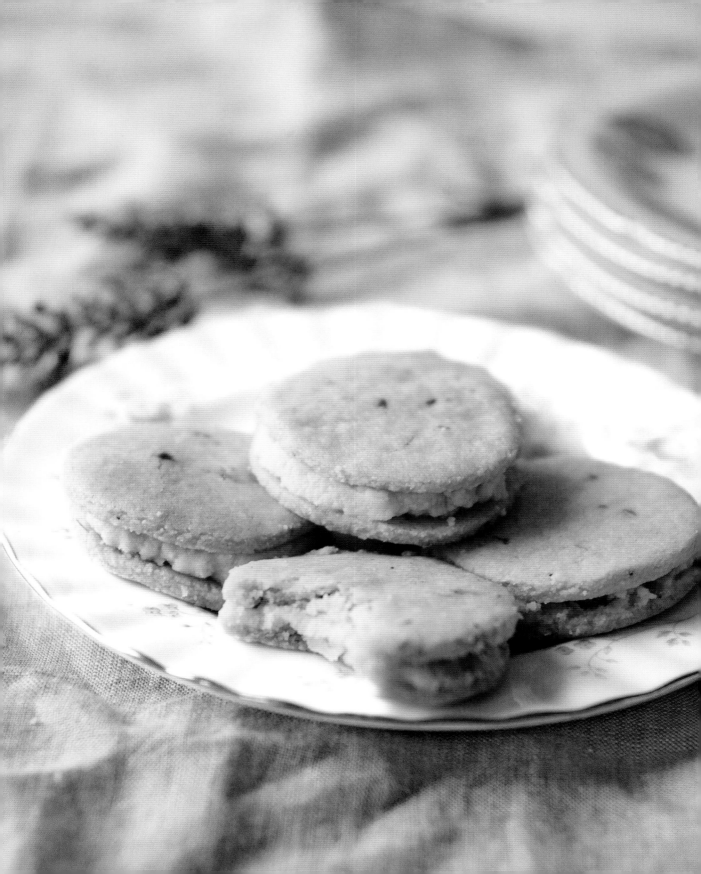

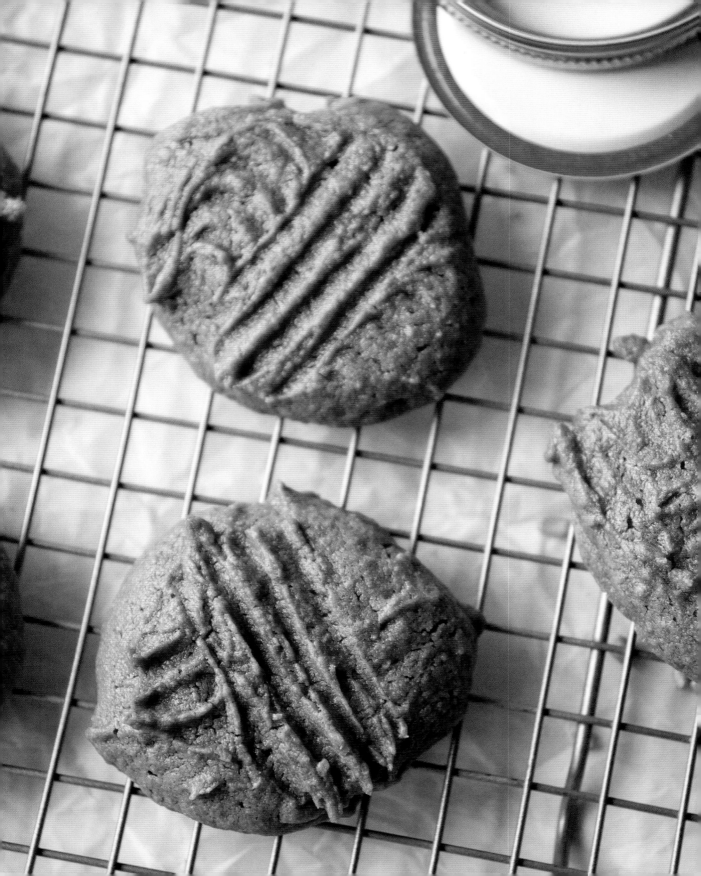

SUNFLOWER SEED BUTTER COOKIES

Crosshatched peanut butter cookies are one of the ultimate classics. However, peanuts are inflammatory for many people, so this recipe keeps the chewy, nutty flavor without the nuts. Sunflower seed butter is creamier and lighter than peanut butter. We're completely addicted to these, and they're perfect for a school bake sale.

MAKES 1 DOZEN COOKIES

1 cup sunflower seed butter

1 large egg

½ cup maple syrup

¾ cup arrowroot powder

½ teaspoon Himalayan pink salt

1 teaspoon vanilla extract

1. Preheat the oven to 350°F. Line a baking sheet with parchment paper.

2. Stir together the sunflower seed butter, egg, maple syrup, arrowroot powder, salt, and vanilla in a medium bowl until a soft dough forms. Using your hands, scoop and roll the dough into 1-inch balls and place on the prepared baking sheet. Transfer to the refrigerator to set for 20 minutes.

3. Use a fork to imprint a crosshatch on each cookie. You may need to dip the fork in some extra arrowroot powder so it doesn't stick to the dough. Bake the cookies for 10 minutes, or until set on top and golden brown on the bottom. Transfer to a rack to cool completely. Store in a sealed container at room temperature for up to 5 days, or in the freezer indefinitely.

CLASSIC SNICKERDOODLES

Growing up, Laurel made cookies for her five brothers on a weekly basis. Usually it was chocolate chip (see page 92), but on special occasions, she made snicker-doodles. Who doesn't love the smell of sweet cinnamon wafting through the air? Chewy and lightly sweet, these cookies are a little piece of perfection. Be sure you have plenty of almond milk on hand for dunking.

MAKES 1 DOZEN LARGE COOKIES

3 cups almond flour

½ teaspoon Himalayan pink salt

½ teaspoon baking soda

2¼ teaspoons ground cinnamon

½ cup coconut oil, melted

½ cup maple syrup

1 tablespoon vanilla extract

¼ cup date sugar (see page 67)

1. Preheat the oven to 350°F. Line a baking sheet with parchment paper.

2. In a large bowl, whisk together the flour, salt, baking soda, and ¼ teaspoon of the cinnamon. In a medium bowl, combine the oil, maple syrup, and vanilla. A little at a time, add the dry ingredients to the wet, stirring until a dough comes together.

3. In a small bowl, mix the date sugar and the remaining 2 teaspoons cinnamon.

4. Place tablespoon-size balls of dough onto the baking sheet and gently press down to flatten to about ¼ inch thick. Sprinkle each cookie with the cinnamon-sugar mixture, then bake for about 10 minutes until golden brown around the edges. Transfer the cookies to a rack to cool slightly—snickerdoodles are best served warm! Store in a sealed container at room temperature for up to 5 days, or in the freezer indefinitely.

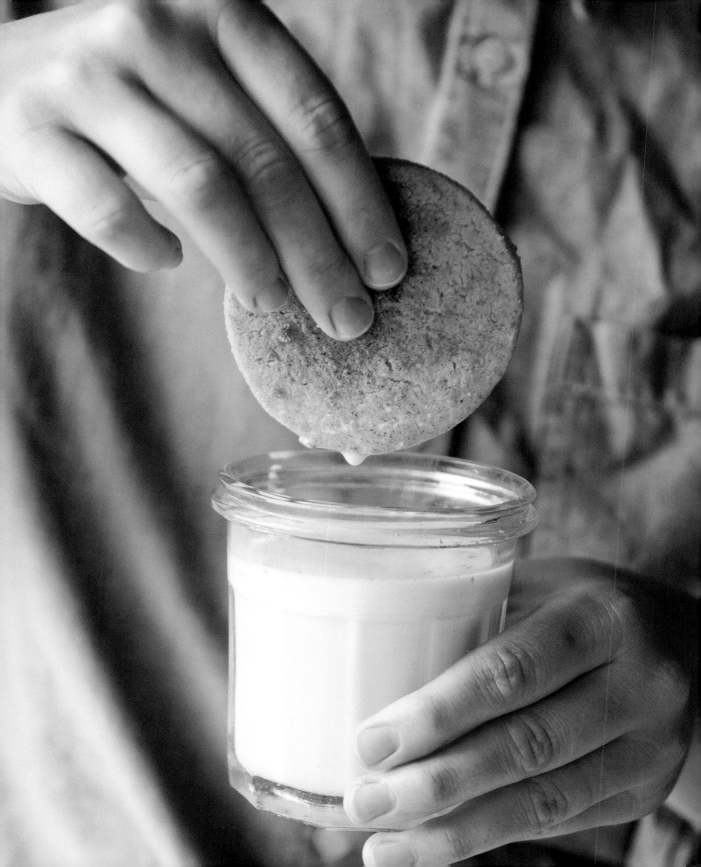

GRAHAM CRACKERS

These crackers started out as a crust for cheesecake—but we liked the crust so much that we found ourselves eating it plain and turned it into its own recipe. Simple, with that classic crunch, these are perfect with maple Marshmallows (page 28) to create s'mores, or even as a snack with a cup of tea.

MAKES 10 CRACKERS

2 cups almond flour

½ cup arrowroot powder

1 teaspoon baking powder

2½ teaspoons ground cinnamon

1½ tablespoons date sugar (see page 67)

¼ teaspoon Himalayan pink salt

3 large egg whites

1 tablespoon coconut oil, melted

1. Preheat the oven to 350°F.

2. In a large bowl, whisk together the flour, arrowroot powder, baking powder, cinnamon, date sugar, and salt. In another large bowl, beat the egg whites until foamy using a hand mixer. A little at a time, fold the egg whites into the dry ingredients, followed by the coconut oil. Stir everything together until a dough forms.

3. Place the dough between two pieces of parchment paper and roll it ¼ inch thick. Remove the top piece of paper and, using a paring knife, cut the dough into rectangles about 5 × 2½ inches. Prick tiny holes on top with a fork.

4. Transfer the crackers and bottom layer of parchment to a baking sheet and bake for 15 minutes, until crisp and golden. Let the crackers rest for at least an hour to cool and set completely, then serve. Store in a sealed container at room temperature for up to 5 days, or in the freezer indefinitely.

FRESH GINGERBREAD COOKIES

The holiday season is not complete without a cozy day in the kitchen dedicated to baking gingerbread. Well, at least that's the way it is in our homes! These festive cookies have the perfect ratio of cinnamon and spice. They're great naked, but we especially love them with our Coconut Buttercream (page 210).

MAKES 1 DOZEN COOKIES

1½ cups almond flour

2 tablespoons arrowroot powder

1 teaspoon baking soda

½ teaspoon Himalayan pink salt

1½ tablespoons ground cinnamon

2 tablespoons grated fresh ginger

¼ cup coconut oil, melted

¼ cup maple syrup

1 tablespoon vanilla extract

1. Preheat the oven to 350°F. Line a baking sheet with parchment paper.

2. In a large bowl, whisk together the flour, arrowroot powder, baking soda, salt, and cinnamon. In a medium bowl, combine the ginger, coconut oil, maple syrup, and vanilla. A little at a time, add the dry ingredients to the wet, stirring until a dough comes together. Gently shape the dough into a ball, cover with plastic wrap, and refrigerate for about 20 minutes.

3. On a large piece of parchment, roll the dough about ¼ inch thick, then cut out desired shapes with cookie cutters and arrange on the baking sheet. Bake for 10 to 15 minutes, until golden brown on the edges. Transfer the cookies to a rack to cool completely. Store in a sealed container at room temperature for up to 5 days, or in the freezer indefinitely.

CHOCOLATE TURTLES

When Claire first created these adorable treats, it was love at first sight for us! Our favorite thing about them is how fancy they look with very little effort. They're now a go-to in both of our homes for a quick and easy dessert. Everyone loves a chocolaty treat complete with gooey caramel, right?

MAKES 1 DOZEN TURTLES

6 ounces 100% cacao unsweetened baking chocolate, melted

2 tablespoons maple syrup

½ teaspoon vanilla extract

1 cup pecan halves, toasted

½ cup Vegan Caramel (page 40), cold

1. In a medium bowl, whisk together the melted cacao, maple syrup, and vanilla.

2. On a sheet of parchment paper, create little mounds of 5 pecans, arranging them to look like the legs of a turtle with a little head poking out. Top each cluster with a tablespoon of cold vegan caramel. Pour the melted cacao over each turtle, letting the pecans (i.e., the legs) stick out a bit.

3. Let the turtles set for at least 30 minutes, until the chocolate is completely hardened. This can be sped up by putting the turtles in the fridge or freezer. Store in a sealed container in the fridge for up to 1 month.

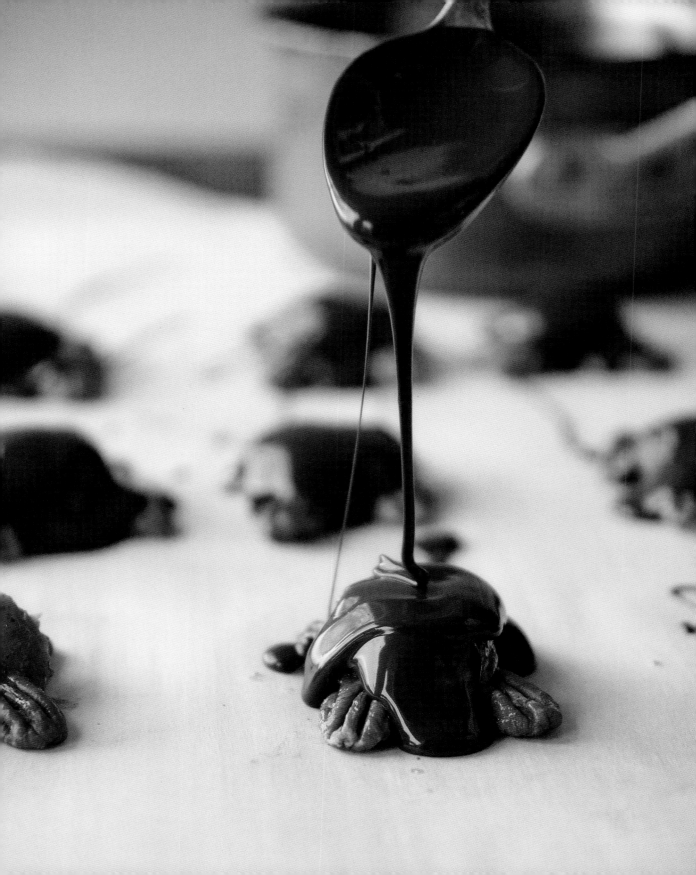

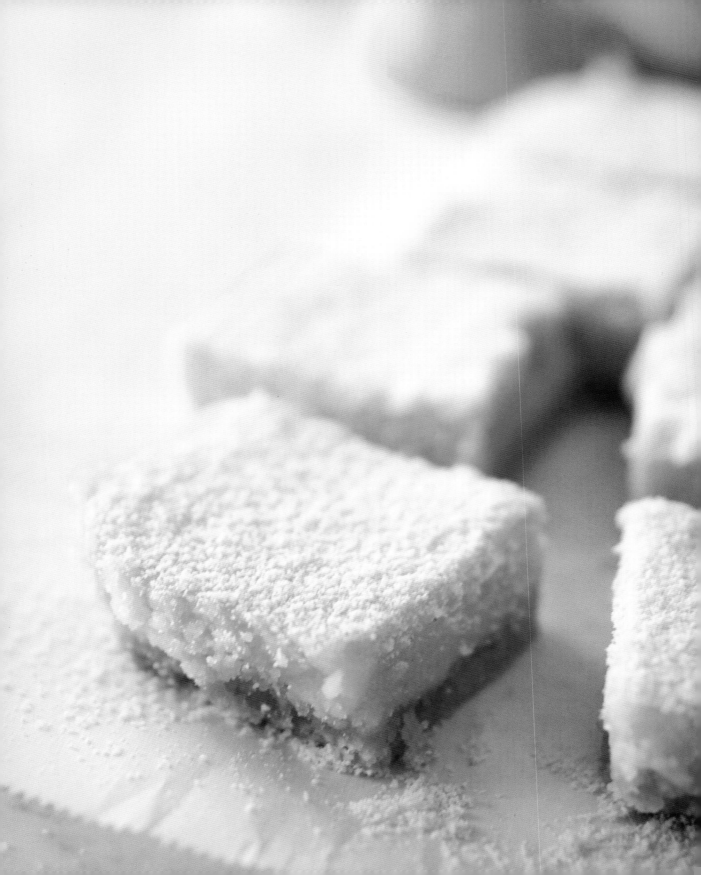

MOM'S LEMON BARS

When Claire was growing up, her mom had a plate of lemon bars on the kitchen table at least once a week. They were so popular, they even made it into Claire's grade school cookbook! The key is balance: not too tart, not too sweet, a tender crust to contrast the creamy lemon curd, and of course an abundance of powdered sugar (or in our case powdered coconut). Now these lemon bars make an appearance on our kitchen tables at least once a week as well.

MAKES 1 DOZEN BARS

FOR THE CRUST

1½ cups almond flour

3 tablespoons coconut oil, melted

2 tablespoons maple syrup

Pinch of Himalayan pink salt

FOR THE FILLING

4 large eggs

¼ cup coconut oil, melted and cooled slightly

⅓ cup honey

½ cup fresh lemon juice

Grated zest of 3 lemons

Shredded Coconut "Powdered Sugar" (page 66), for serving

1. Preheat the oven to 350°F. Line an 8 × 8-inch pan with parchment paper, letting the paper hang over the sides for easy removal.

2. **MAKE THE CRUST:** Whisk together the flour, coconut oil, maple syrup, and salt in a medium bowl until a soft dough forms. Press the dough into the bottom of the prepared pan, about ¼ inch thick, and bake for 15 minutes until just golden brown on the edges. Remove from the oven and allow the crust to cool while you make the filling.

3. **MAKE THE FILLING:** In the bowl of a stand mixer fitted with the whisk attachment, whip the eggs for about 4 minutes, until frothy. Slowly add the coconut oil and honey, and mix until combined. Fold in the lemon juice and zest by hand. Before adding the filling to the cooled crust, let the filling settle so there are no bubbles on top. You can tap the bowl of filling on your counter a few times to help pop any bubbles.

4. Pour the filling into the cooled crust and bake for another 15 to 25 minutes, or until set at the edges and just barely jiggling at the center. Let the bars cool and set completely in the pan, then dust with "powdered sugar" and cut into squares. Store in a sealed container at room temperature for up to 3 days.

APPLE PIE BARS

We're so into apple pie. The flavors, the smell, the ooey-gooey appley-ness. Especially with a big scoop of melting vanilla ice cream . . . The first time we made these bars, we couldn't stop eating the filling. But paired with this flaky crust, crunchy streusel, and caramel, these bars are beyond delicious.

MAKES 1 DOZEN BARS

FOR THE CRUST

2 cups almond flour

½ teaspoon Himalayan pink salt

2 tablespoons coconut oil, melted

1 large egg

FOR THE FILLING

5 to 7 tart apples, such as Pink Lady or Honeycrisp, peeled, cored, and sliced

2 tablespoons maple syrup

1 teaspoon ground cinnamon

Juice of 1 lemon

1 tablespoon coconut oil, solid

FOR THE STREUSEL TOPPING

1 cup almond flour

2 tablespoons coconut oil, melted

¼ cup maple syrup

1 teaspoon ground cinnamon

1 cup Vegan Caramel (page 40), for serving

1. Preheat the oven to 350°F. Line a 13 × 9-inch pan with parchment paper, letting the paper hang over the edges for easy removal.

2. **MAKE THE CRUST:** In a medium bowl, whisk together the flour and salt, then gradually stir in the coconut oil and egg. Mix well until everything is incorporated and a soft dough forms. Press the dough into the bottom of the prepared pan and set aside.

3. **MAKE THE FILLING:** In a large bowl, combine the apples, maple syrup, cinnamon, and lemon juice. Mix to coat the apples thoroughly. Melt the coconut oil in a large heavy-duty saucepan over medium heat. Add the apple mixture to the pan and sauté for 5 to 10 minutes, until syrupy. Remove the pan from the heat and allow the mixture to cool slightly. Arrange the coated apple slices in rows across the crust, pouring any leftover pan liquid over them. Bake the bars for 40 to 50 minutes, until the apple slices are golden brown and tender but not mushy.

4. **MAKE THE STREUSEL TOPPING:** In a medium bowl, whisk together the flour, coconut oil, maple syrup, and cinnamon and stir until a batter forms. Sprinkle the streusel over the cooked apples and return the bars to the oven. Bake for 10 minutes, or until the streusel turns golden brown, then remove from the oven. Holding two sides of the parchment, lift the bars in one piece from the pan; allow to cool slightly on a rack. Before serving, drizzle the caramel sauce over the bars and cut into squares. Store in a sealed container at room temperature for up to 3 days.

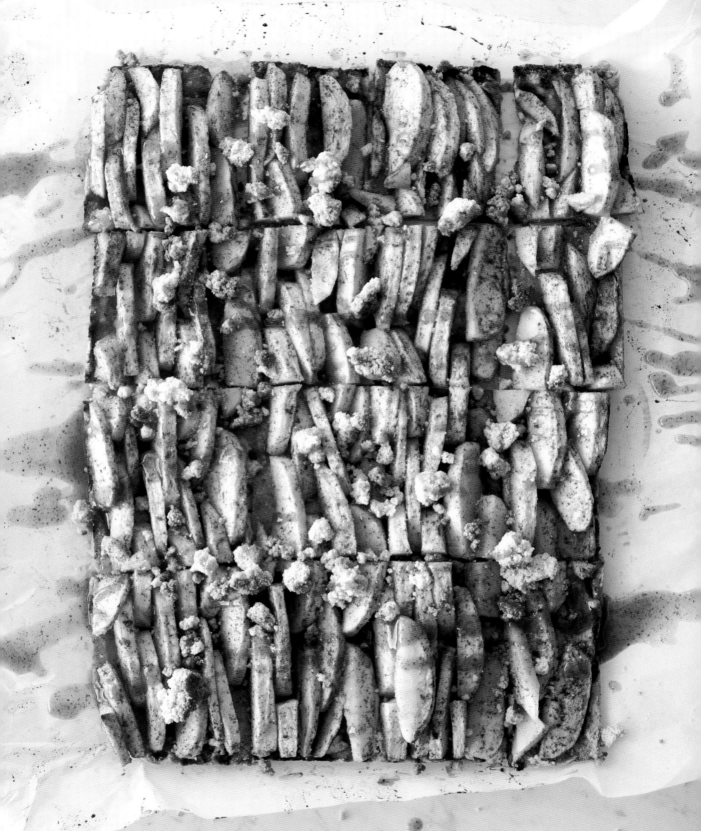

DOUBLE CHOCOLATE BROWNIES

People go nuts when we tell them these brownies are gluten- and dairy-free. Imagine if a sticky toffee pudding and a brownie had a baby—yep, delicious. Warm, gooey, rich, tender, crumbly, glass-of-almond-milk-inducing wonderfulness—you really should go make some. Like, now.

MAKES 1 DOZEN BROWNIES

2 cups almond butter, store-bought or homemade (page 38)

2 large eggs

1¼ cups maple syrup

1 tablespoon vanilla extract

½ cup 100% unsweetened cacao powder

1 teaspoon baking soda

½ teaspoon Himalayan pink salt

1 cup vegan chocolate chips, store-bought or homemade (page 42)

1. Preheat the oven to 350°F. Line an 8 × 8-inch pan with parchment paper, letting it hang over the sides for easy removal.

2. In the bowl of a stand mixer fitted with the paddle attachment, mix the almond butter on medium speed, then mix in the eggs, one at a time, maple syrup, and vanilla. In a medium bowl, whisk together the cacao powder, baking soda, and salt. A little at a time, add the dry ingredients to the wet, stirring until a dough comes together. Stir in about three-fourths of the chocolate chips, then pour the batter into the prepared pan.

3. Sprinkle the remaining chocolate chips over the top of the brownies and bake for 35 to 40 minutes, until set on the edges and still a bit fudgy in the center, then remove from the oven. Holding two sides of the parchment, lift the brownies in one piece from the pan; allow to cool slightly on a rack before cutting into squares. Store in a sealed container at room temperature for up to 5 days, or in the freezer indefinitely.

HOMEMADE ICE CREAM CONES

One of our favorite grain-free discoveries came on the day Laurel created these delicious ice cream cones. Crunchy and crisp are two of the harder textures to achieve in refined-sugar-free baking. Sugar hardens as it caramelizes and gives structure to anything it's in, so achieving a perfect ice cream cone without it was a challenge. Laurel experimented on the pizzelle maker her in-laws had given her, and these simple, addictive cones were the result. We even love these as flat, crisp cookies—perfect served with fresh fruit and a little raw honey!

**MAKES 6 SMALL CONES
OR 3 LARGE CONES**

⅔ cup almond flour

Pinch of Himalayan pink salt

2 large eggs

2 tablespoons maple syrup

2 tablespoons coconut oil, melted, plus more for greasing the iron

1 teaspoon vanilla extract

1. Preheat a waffle iron or pizzelle maker.

2. In a medium bowl, whisk together the flour, salt, eggs, maple syrup, coconut oil, and vanilla until smooth and well blended.

3. Just before cooking, lightly grease the iron with coconut oil. Place 1 tablespoon batter in the center of the iron. Close the iron and cook until golden brown, about 2 minutes. For large cones, use 2 tablespoons of batter.

4. Remove and roll into a cone. The handle of an ice cream scooper works well as a cone guide. The waffle is hot, so either work quickly or use a tea towel to protect your fingertips as you shape the cone. Repeat with the remaining batter and make the rest of the cones.

5. Let the cones cool completely to harden. This happens pretty quickly, so we just let the cones cool on the counter. They should be quite crisp. If making them in advance, keep them uncovered for up to 2 days. If they get soft, crisp them up by placing them in a 350°F oven for 10 minutes.

Notes

To make our cones, we use a pizzelle maker, but any waffle cone iron will work as well. A standard round waffle iron (not Belgian style) works, too, but the cones may be on the thicker side.

We mold the cones by hand, but you can use a cone roller for an easier, quicker process.

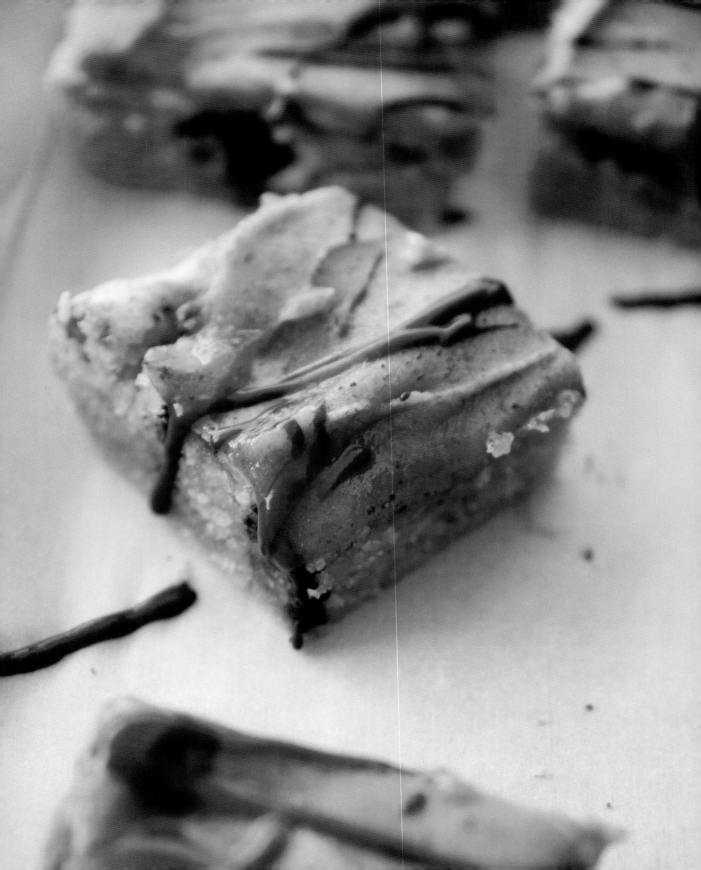

CHOCOLATE CARAMEL BLONDIES

Chewy, rich, caramel-filled . . . sounds pretty great, right? So there should be no excuses for all of the lame blondie recipes out there. A blondie is not a lesser brownie; a blondie is like a brownie with a tan. There are so many delicious things happening in these golden little bars, making them a great alternative for when you've maxed out on brownies. We know—sounds unbelievable, but trust us, it can happen.

MAKES 1 DOZEN BARS

3 cups almond flour

¼ cup coconut oil, melted

¼ cup maple syrup

3 tablespoons vanilla extract

Pinch of Himalayan pink salt

1 cup vegan chocolate chips, store-bought or homemade (page 42)

1 cup Vegan Caramel (page 40)

1. Preheat the oven to 350°F. Line an 8 × 8-inch pan with parchment paper, letting it hang over the sides for easy removal.

2. In a large bowl, combine the flour, coconut oil, maple syrup, vanilla, and salt. Stir until a dough comes together, then add ½ cup of the chocolate chips. Press the dough into the bottom of the prepared pan.

3. Bake for 12 to 15 minutes, until firm but not quite golden. Remove from the oven and, holding two sides of the parchment, lift the blondies in one piece from the pan. Transfer to a rack to cool completely. Pour the caramel evenly over the blondies, and let set. If it's warm out, set the blondies in the fridge to help the caramel firm up.

4. To make the chocolate drizzle, melt the remaining ½ cup chocolate chips in a glass bowl, either in a microwave (zap for 15-second increments on low power, stirring in between) or in a double boiler (see Note, page 48). Use a spoon to drizzle the melted chocolate over the blondies and let set. Once the drizzle is set, cut the blondies into squares and serve. Store in a sealed container at room temperature for up to 5 days, or in the freezer indefinitely.

HELLO DOLLY LAYER BARS

Laurel was the Hello Dolly queen in high school. At every bake sale, she would whip up these decadent bars, and they would sell out in minutes. You might know these as magic bars or layer bars, but whatever you call them, we're sure you know they're delicious. Using the same classic layers, but with wholesome ingredients, Hello Dollies are getting a makeover while keeping all of their fabulous flavor.

MAKES 1 DOZEN BARS

1½ cups almond flour

3 tablespoons coconut oil, melted

2 tablespoons maple syrup

¼ teaspoon Himalayan pink salt

2 cups vegan chocolate chips, store-bought or homemade (page 42)

1 cup finely chopped pecans

½ cup full-fat coconut milk

1 tablespoon arrowroot powder

4 Medjool dates or ¼ cup date paste, store-bought or homemade (page 42)

2 cups unsweetened shredded coconut

1. Preheat the oven to 350°F. Line an 8 × 8-inch pan with parchment paper, letting the paper hang over the sides for easy removal.

2. Combine the flour, coconut oil, maple syrup, and salt in a medium bowl and stir until a dough forms. Press the dough into the bottom of the prepared pan.

3. Cover the first layer completely with the chocolate chips, followed by the chopped pecans.

4. In a food processor, combine the coconut milk, arrowroot powder, and dates until completely incorporated. Spread the mixture into the pan, then top with shredded coconut. Bake for 30 minutes or until everything is set and the coconut is lightly toasted. Holding two sides of the parchment, lift the bars in one piece from the pan; allow to cool slightly on a rack before cutting into squares. Store in a sealed container at room temperature for up to 5 days, or in the freezer indefinitely.

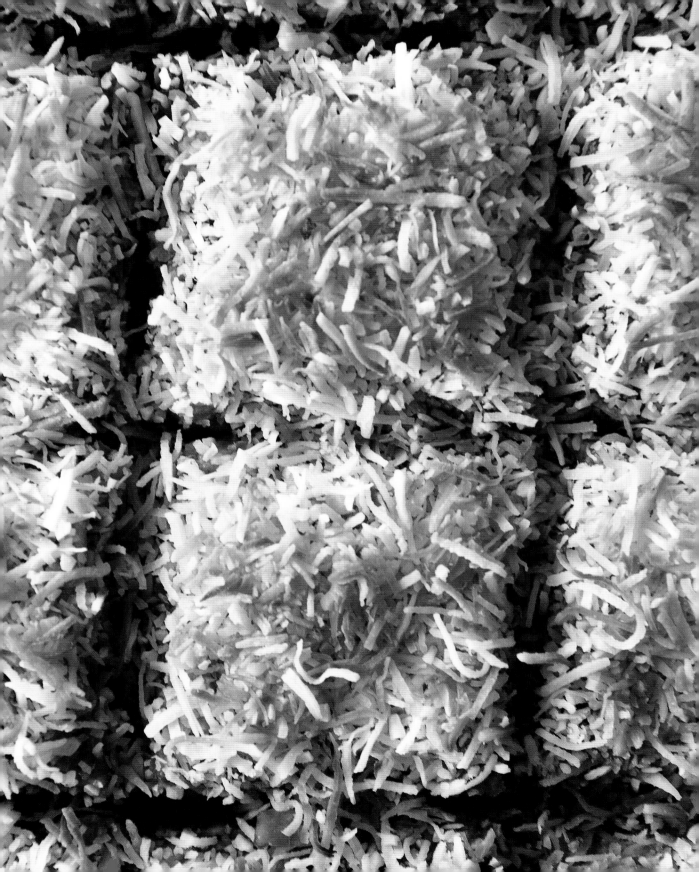

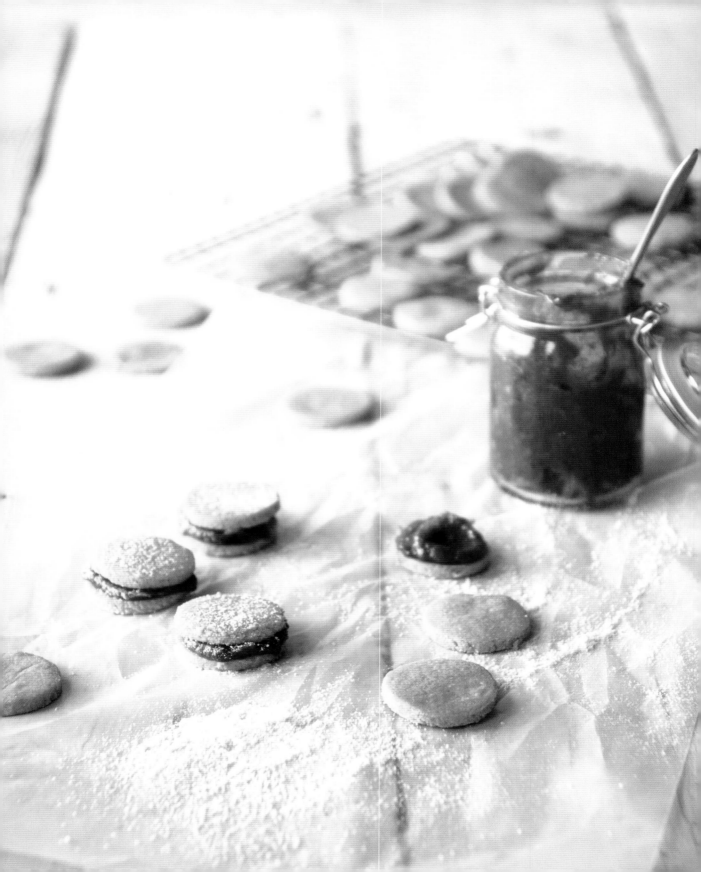

ALFAJORES

Our favorite coffee shop is just blocks from where we grew up, and one of its featured treats is the *alfajore*, a melt-in-your-mouth Argentinian sandwich cookie. Traditionally made with shortbread, dulce de leche, and an abundance of powdered sugar, it's the perfect cookie to pair with a cup of strong South American coffee. In our version, we switch out the dulce de leche for our vegan caramel, and coat the cookies in our coconut powdered sugar. Don't forget to brew a pot of coffee!

MAKES 18 SANDWICH COOKIES

2 cups almond flour

⅛ teaspoon Himalayan pink salt

¼ cup coconut oil, melted

¼ cup maple syrup

Shredded Coconut "Powdered Sugar" (page 66), for topping

Vegan Caramel (page 40), for filling

1. Preheat the oven to 350°F. Line a baking sheet with parchment paper.

2. In a medium bowl, whisk together the flour and salt. In a small bowl, combine the coconut oil and maple syrup. A little at a time, add the dry ingredients to the wet, stirring until a dough comes together.

3. Place the dough between two pieces of parchment paper and roll it about ⅛ inch thick. Remove the top piece of paper and, using a 1½-inch round cookie cutter, cut the dough into circles and place on the prepared baking sheet. Bake for 7 to 9 minutes, until the edges begin turning golden brown. Transfer the cookies to a rack, dust heavily with "powdered sugar," and cool completely while you prepare the vegan caramel.

4. Gently spread 1 to 2 teaspoons of vegan caramel onto a cooled cookie, then sandwich together with another cookie. Repeat with the remaining cookies and serve. Store in a sealed container at room temperature for up to 5 days, or in the freezer indefinitely.

GOOEY CAST-IRON COOKIE

A gooey, warm cookie topped with ice cream is one of our favorite desserts. It just always manages to hit the spot. But in our style of baking, it's not as simple as putting just any cookie dough in a pan and underbaking it. To get a deep, caramelized brown sugar flavor and spoonable texture, we added plenty of date paste, maple syrup, and almond butter. This recipe is based on a classic chocolate chip cookie, but you can add whatever fillings and garnishes you like: nuts, marshmallows, the works!

MAKES ONE 9-INCH PAN COOKIE

¼ cup coconut oil, melted, plus more for greasing the pan

2½ cups almond flour

½ cup maple syrup

⅓ cup date paste, store-bought or homemade (page 42)

½ cup almond butter, store-bought or homemade (page 38)

2 large eggs

3 tablespoons vanilla extract

½ teaspoon Himalayan pink salt

1 cup vegan chocolate chips, store-bought or homemade (page 42)

Creamy Dairy-Free Ice Cream (page 228), for serving

1. Preheat the oven to 350°F. Grease a 9-inch cast-iron pan with coconut oil.

2. In a large bowl, combine the coconut oil, flour, maple syrup, date paste, almond butter, eggs, vanilla, and salt. Stir well until a dough comes together, then add ½ cup of the chocolate chips. Press the dough into the bottom of the prepared pan.

3. Bake for 15 to 20 minutes, until golden and firm at the edges (the middle will still be a bit gooey). Remove from the oven, garnish with the remaining chocolate chips and ice cream, and devour while still warm in the pan you baked it in.

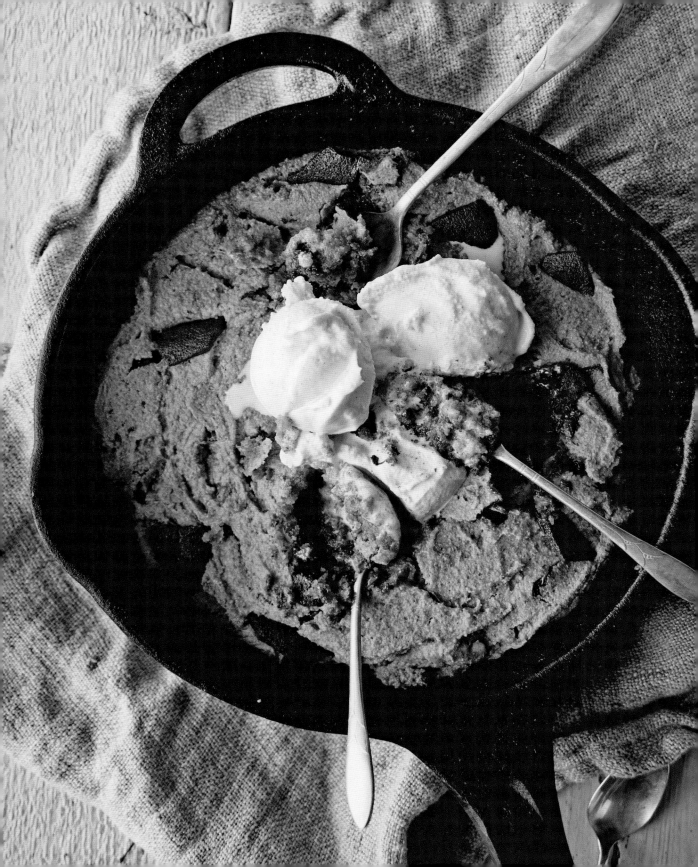

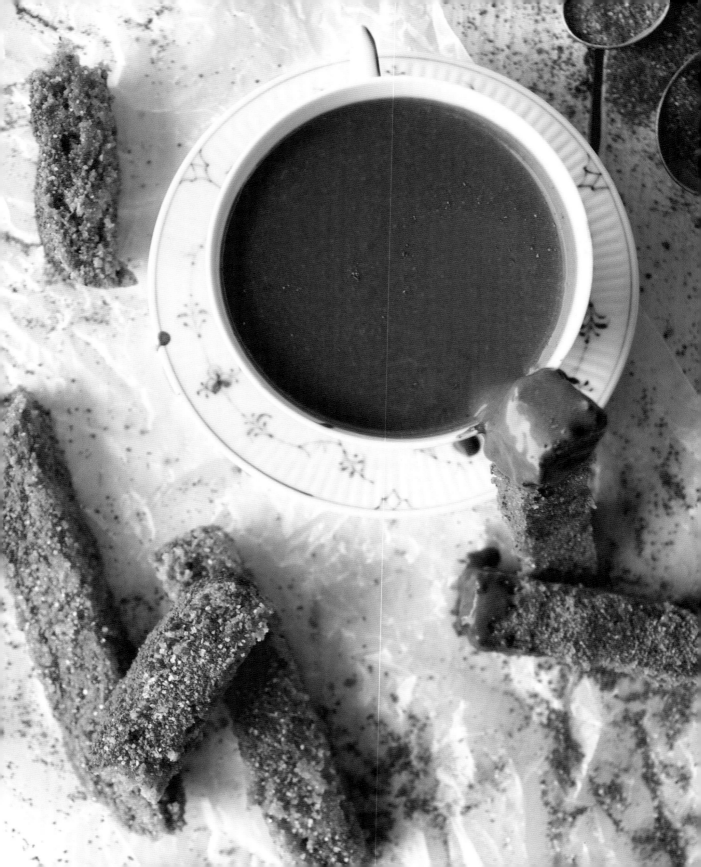

BAKED CHURRO BARS

We know churros as the foot-and-a-half-long doughnuts we devour with sticky fingers at carnivals or amusement parks, but the true version of a churro is a little bit more refined. In Spain and Mexico, they're served with rich drinking chocolate, which is essentially melted chocolate with a touch of cream. You dunk the churro into the chocolate, crumbs of cinnamon sugar accidentally swirling in, and get a gorgeous combination of textures and flavors. Crunchy, warm, sweet, and a little gooey, it's all totally indulgent and delicious. This combination inspired these delicious churro bars—cinnamon and pecan-flecked cake, coated in cinnamon date sugar. Serve with a steaming cup of melted cacao or enjoy the bars alone.

MAKES 16 BARS AND 1½ CUPS DIPPING CHOCOLATE

FOR THE TOPPING

¼ cup date sugar (see page 67)

1 tablespoon ground cinnamon

FOR THE CAKE

3 cups almond flour

1 teaspoon baking soda

½ teaspoon Himalayan pink salt

½ cup finely chopped pecans or pecan flour

2 large eggs

½ cup maple syrup

½ cup coconut oil, melted

1 tablespoon vanilla extract

FOR THE DIPPING CACAO (OPTIONAL)

½ cup chopped 100% cacao unsweetened baking chocolate

1 cup full-fat coconut milk

¼ cup maple syrup

1 teaspoon vanilla extract

Pinch of Himalayan pink salt

1. Preheat the oven to 350°F. Line an 8 × 8-inch baking pan with parchment paper, letting the paper hang over the sides for easy removal.

2. **MAKE THE TOPPING:** Mix the date sugar and cinnamon together in a small bowl and set aside.

3. **MAKE THE CAKE:** In a medium bowl, mix the flour, baking soda, salt, and pecans. In a large bowl, mix the eggs, maple syrup, coconut oil, and vanilla. Pour the dry ingredients into the wet, stirring to combine. Pour the batter into the prepared baking pan. Sprinkle with the cinnamon date sugar and bake for 30 to 35 minutes, until golden brown and a toothpick inserted into the center comes out clean.

4. Allow the cake to cool fully in the pan. Remove the cake from the pan by gently lifting up on the parchment paper, then cut into thin slices, about the size of churros, 1 × 4 inches. Sprinkle with additional date sugar if you like.

5. To serve with drinking chocolate, combine the cacao, coconut milk, maple syrup, vanilla, and salt in a small pot over low heat. Stir gently until everything is melted, steaming, and well combined, about 10 minutes. Pour into 4 cups to sip with the churro bars (it's decadent drinking chocolate, so a little goes a long way).

ROCKY ROAD COOKIES

Chocolate, marshmallows, and nuts are a perfect combination. There's depth and a touch of bitterness from the chocolate, the marshmallows are fluffy and perfectly sweet, and the nuts add some much-needed crunch. We're used to seeing these ingredients striped through a quart of ice cream, but here we feature them as delicious cookies. Our favorite part is how the marshmallows caramelize and crisp at the edges when baked, adding a hint of toffee flavor.

MAKES 16 COOKIES

⅔ cup date paste, store-bought or homemade (page 42)

¼ cup maple syrup

⅓ cup coconut oil, melted

1 tablespoon vanilla extract

2 cups almond flour

¼ teaspoon baking soda

¼ teaspoon Himalayan pink salt

¼ cup 100% unsweetened cacao powder

⅓ cup arrowroot powder

⅔ cup chopped marshmallows, store-bought or homemade (page 28)

⅔ cup roughly chopped walnuts

1 cup vegan chocolate chips, store-bought or homemade (page 42)

1. Preheat the oven to 350°F. Line a baking sheet with parchment paper.

2. In a food processor, pulse the date paste, maple syrup, coconut oil, and vanilla until blended. In a medium bowl, whisk together the flour, baking soda, salt, cacao powder, and arrowroot powder. A little at a time, add the dry ingredients to the date paste mixture, pulsing until a dough forms.

3. Transfer the dough to a sheet of parchment. Knead the marshmallows, walnuts, and ½ cup of the chocolate chips into the dough and gradually form it into a ball. Roll the ball into a 2½-inch-thick log. Wrap the log in plastic and refrigerate for 30 minutes to set the dough.

4. Cut the dough into ½-inch slices. Place the slices on the baking sheet about 2 inches apart. Bake for 9 to 10 minutes, until the edges are fully set, then transfer the cookies to a rack to cool completely.

5. To make the chocolate drizzle, melt the remaining ½ cup chocolate chips in a glass bowl either for 10 seconds in a microwave or over a pot of boiling water. Use a spoon to drizzle the melted chocolate over each cookie. Let the drizzle set, then serve. Store any leftovers in a sealed container no longer than 3 days for ideal freshness. These also freeze well indefinitely.

Note

These cookies can be made in the traditional "drop" fashion, where spoonfuls are mounded and dropped on the cookie sheet, but we prefer rolling the dough into a log and making thick slices. It creates a larger, fudgier cookie.

ORANGE CHAI SHORTBREAD

Our layer cakes and pies tend to get all of the attention, but this cookie recipe is one of our understated favorites. Every year Claire hosts a holiday cookie swap with all of her girlfriends, and every year Laurel brings a platter of grain-free loveliness. One year, these orange chai shortbreads hit the table and were cleaned out before half the crowd had even arrived. Their light sweetness isn't cloying, the orange is vibrant and bright, and the spices aren't overpowering—the black pepper and fennel add an unexpected earthiness.

MAKES 2 DOZEN COOKIES

2 cups almond flour

¼ teaspoon Himalayan pink salt

¼ teaspoon ground cardamom

¼ teaspoon ground black pepper

¼ teaspoon ground fennel

½ teaspoon ground ginger

½ teaspoon ground cinnamon, plus more for garnish

¼ cup coconut oil, melted

⅓ cup maple syrup

2 teaspoons grated orange zest

1 teaspoon vanilla extract

Orange Coconut Glaze (page 221), for garnish

1. Preheat the oven to 350°F. Line a baking sheet with parchment paper.

2. In a large bowl, whisk together the flour, salt, cardamom, pepper, fennel, ginger, and cinnamon. In a medium bowl, whisk the coconut oil, maple syrup, orange zest, and vanilla. A little at a time, add the dry ingredients to the wet, stirring until a dough comes together.

3. Place the dough between two pieces of parchment paper and roll it about ⅛ inch thick. Remove the top piece of paper and, using a 2-inch round cookie cutter, cut the dough into circles and place on the prepared baking sheet. Bake for 9 to 10 minutes, until the edges begin turning golden brown. Transfer the cookies to a rack to cool completely while you prepare the glaze.

4. Gently spread 1 to 2 teaspoons of orange coconut glaze onto each cooled cookie, then sprinkle with a little cinnamon. Store in a sealed container at room temperature for up to 5 days, or in the freezer indefinitely.

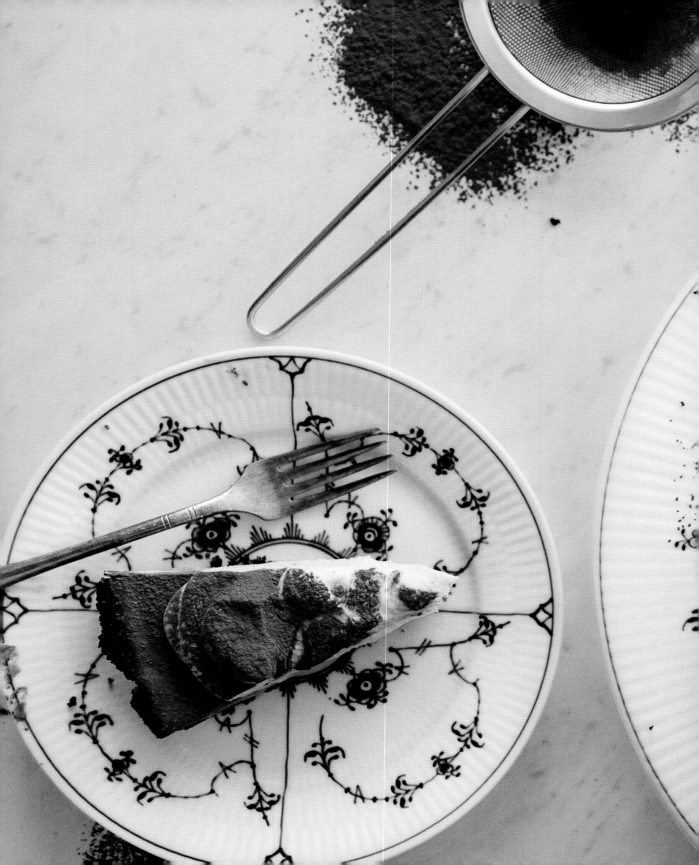

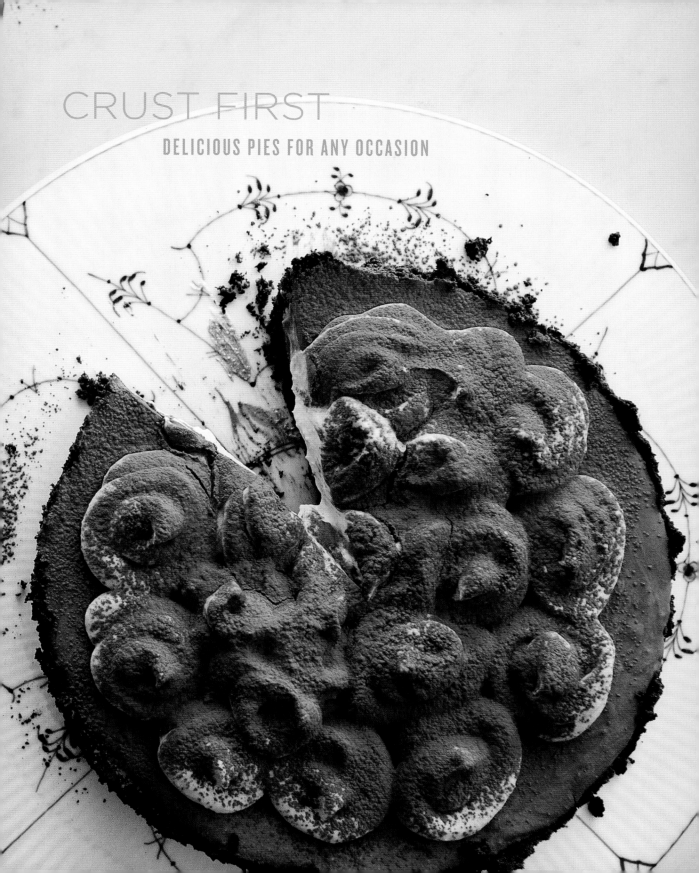

CRUST FIRST

DELICIOUS PIES FOR ANY OCCASION

DARK CHOCOLATE CHIFFON PIE

Chocolate on chocolate with whipped cream . . . how could that be a bad thing? This rich chocolate pie is one of our most elegant recipes. It's also one of the most intense in flavor, so remember, a small slice goes a long way. We love this served with espresso after dinner—or straight out of the fridge after midnight.

MAKES ONE 9-INCH PIE

FOR THE CRUST

¼ cup coconut oil, melted, plus more for greasing the pan

2¼ cups Brazil nuts or hazelnuts

3 tablespoons date paste, store-bought or homemade (page 42)

¼ teaspoon Himalayan pink salt

½ cup 100% unsweetened cacao powder

FOR THE FILLING

3 cups full-fat coconut milk

2 teaspoons gelatin powder

4 large egg yolks

⅓ cup maple syrup

1 teaspoon vanilla extract

2 ounces 100% cacao unsweetened baking chocolate, roughly chopped

2 tablespoons 100% unsweetened cacao powder

¼ teaspoon Himalayan pink salt

4 cups Coconut Whipped Cream (page 30)

2 tablespoons 100% unsweetened cacao powder, for topping

1. Preheat the oven to 350°F. Generously grease a 9-inch pie pan with coconut oil.

2. **MAKE THE CRUST:** Combine the nuts, coconut oil, date paste, salt, and cacao powder in a food processor and pulse until the mixture forms a ball. Lightly press the dough into the pie pan and bake for 10 to 12 minutes, until fragrant and set. Set aside to cool.

3. **MAKE THE FILLING:** Pour the coconut milk into a small saucepan and sprinkle the gelatin on top. Allow the gelatin to soften for about 5 minutes. In a medium bowl, whisk together the egg yolks, maple syrup, and vanilla.

4. Whisk the coconut milk and gelatin over low heat until smooth and warm. Add 1 cup of the warm coconut milk mixture to the egg yolk mixture, stirring constantly. Pour the entire yolk mixture into the saucepan and mix well. Add the chopped cacao, cacao powder, and salt. Whisking constantly, bring the mixture to a simmer and cook for 3 to 5 minutes, until thickened. Transfer the filling to a bowl and refrigerate until cool but not quite set, about 40 minutes

5. Fold 2 cups of the coconut whipped cream into the filling, then pour the filling into the crust and refrigerate overnight, or for at least 8 hours.

6. Top with the remaining whipped coconut cream and sift the cacao powder over the pie. Serve immediately or refrigerate for up to 2 days.

Note

The chocolate custard filling needs to set overnight, so be sure to plan ahead.

S'MORES PIE

What is it that makes burnt things taste so good? OK, burnt pizza, maybe not, but burnt sugar? Definitely yes. Combining smooth, rich chocolate and a lightly spiced graham cracker crust, this pie is one of our favorites. It also was one of the biggest challenges to create. We'd had great success making marshmallows with honey, but the moment we started toasting them, they'd melt away instead of caramelize. We pivoted to maple syrup after learning about its ability to caramelize and turn into hard toffee, and our toasted marshmallow problems were solved. The chocolate custard filling needs to set overnight, so be sure to plan ahead.

MAKES ONE 9-INCH PIE

FOR THE CRUST

6 Graham Crackers
(page 104)

3 tablespoons coconut
oil, melted

Pinch of Himalayan
pink salt

2 tablespoons maple
syrup

FOR THE FILLING

2 cups full-fat coconut
milk

2 teaspoons gelatin
powder

4 large egg yolks

½ cup maple syrup

1 teaspoon vanilla extract

2 ounces 100% cacao
unsweetened baking
chocolate, roughly
chopped

2 tablespoons
100% unsweetened
cacao powder

¼ teaspoon
Himalayan pink salt

1. Preheat the oven to 350°F.

2. **MAKE THE CRUST:** Pulse together the graham crackers, coconut oil, salt, and maple syrup in a food processor until the mixture reaches a wet sand consistency. Gently press the dough into the pie pan and bake for 10 to 12 minutes, until fragrant and deep golden brown. Allow to cool completely. This can be done up to 3 days in advance.

3. **MAKE THE FILLING:** Pour the coconut milk into a small saucepan and sprinkle the gelatin on top. Allow the gelatin to soften for about 5 minutes. In a medium bowl, whisk together the egg yolks, maple syrup, and vanilla.

4. Whisk the coconut milk and gelatin mixture over low heat until smooth and warm, about 5 minutes. Add a cup of the warm coconut milk, between 90°F and 100°F, to the egg yolk mixture and stir constantly. Then pour the entire yolk mixture into the saucepan and mix well. Add the cacao, cacao powder, and salt and cook, whisking constantly, until the chocolate has melted and the ingredients are warmed through, about 10 minutes. Pour the mixture into the cooled crust and refrigerate overnight, or for at least 8 hours.

(RECIPE CONTINUES)

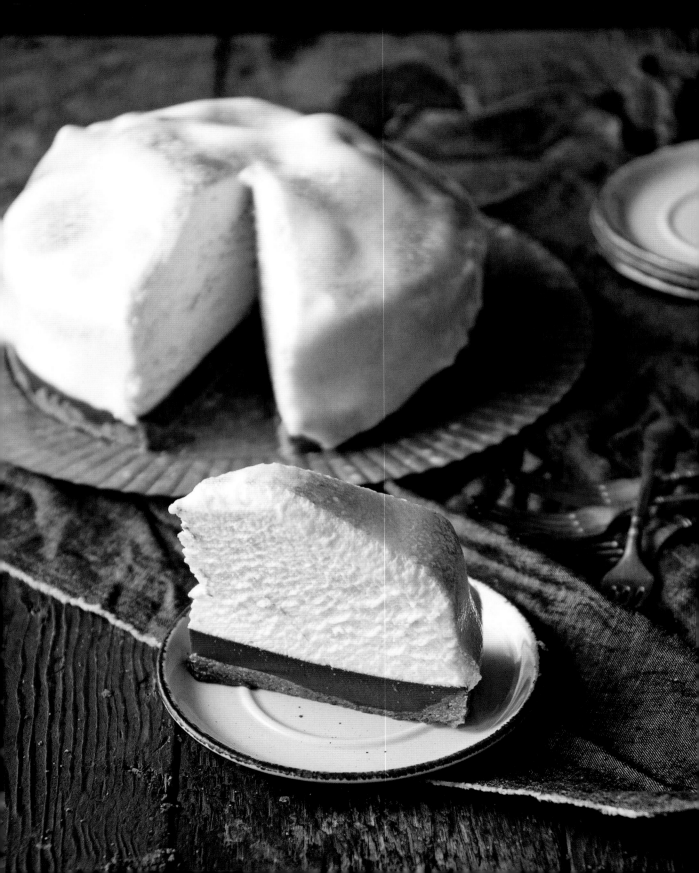

FOR THE TOPPING

3 tablespoons gelatin powder

1 cup maple syrup

1 teaspoon vanilla extract

¼ teaspoon Himalayan pink salt

5. **MAKE THE TOPPING:** In the bowl of a stand mixer fitted with the whisk attachment, pour in ½ cup water and sprinkle the gelatin on top. Let soften for about 5 minutes.

6. In a medium saucepan over medium heat, combine ½ cup water, the maple syrup, and vanilla. Bring the mixture to a simmer and use a candy thermometer to monitor the temperature until it reaches 240°F. Remove the pan from the heat.

7. With the mixer on medium-high speed, blend the gelatin and water. Slowly pour in the syrup and continue to beat for about 10 minutes, until the steam disappears and soft peaks form. Don't let it sit, as the marshmallow topping will set and get stiff.

8. Immediately spoon the marshmallow over the pie filling, mounding it in the middle. Let the marshmallow topping set for about an hour at room temperature. Then, if desired, toast the peaks of the marshmallow topping with a butane torch or (very carefully) singe them under your broiler. This pie is best served the day it's made. It will keep in the fridge for up to 2 days, though we like the marshmallows toasted just before serving.

Note

We love this recipe as a showstopping pie, but you can easily turn it into a personal s'mores jar—just put the finished crust, crumbled, in the bottom of each jar, and add the chocolate custard filling and marshmallow topping as dictated in the recipe.

THE BEST PECAN PIE

When she was in middle school, Laurel's job was to make twelve pies for family Thanksgiving. It sounds like a lot, but considering that her nuclear family is nine people deep, when you add in-laws, cousins, and children, twelve is about right. Laurel was always shocked by the amount of corn syrup required for pecan pie. When our first Thanksgiving at Sweet Laurel came around, she was determined to make ours taste just as good, but without the corn syrup. By combining dates and maple syrup, our pecan pie filling is richer, more caramelized, and more intense (in a good way) than a conventional pecan pie, and it has completely replaced the bad stuff on the Thanksgiving table. It's so good that one of our customers even has a standing order for her weekly pecan pie over the holidays!

MAKES ONE 9-INCH PIE

FOR THE CRUST

¼ cup coconut oil, solid, plus more for greasing the pan

2½ cups almond flour

1 cup arrowroot powder

¼ cup maple syrup

1 large egg

Pinch of Himalayan pink salt

FOR THE FILLING

¾ cup maple syrup

1 cup date paste, store-bought or homemade (page 42)

3 large eggs

¼ cup coconut oil, melted

1 tablespoon vanilla extract

1 teaspoon Himalayan pink salt

4 cups pecan halves

1. Preheat the oven to 350°F. Grease a 9-inch pie pan with coconut oil.

2. **MAKE THE CRUST:** Combine all the crust ingredients in a large bowl and mix with a pastry blender or your fingertips until a dough comes together. It will look like wet sand, and the fats should be pea sized. Gently shape the dough into a ball, cover with plastic wrap, and chill in the freezer for about an hour.

3. **MAKE THE FILLING:** In a blender or food processor, pulse together the maple syrup and date paste until combined. Add the eggs, coconut oil, vanilla, and salt and blend well. Transfer to a large bowl and gently stir in the pecans.

4. Roll out the dough ¼ inch thick, then place in the prepared pan and trim any excess. Pour the filling into the crust. Bake for 30 to 35 minutes, until the center of the pie is firm. Serve slightly warm. Store in a sealed container in the fridge for up to 5 days, or in the freezer indefinitely.

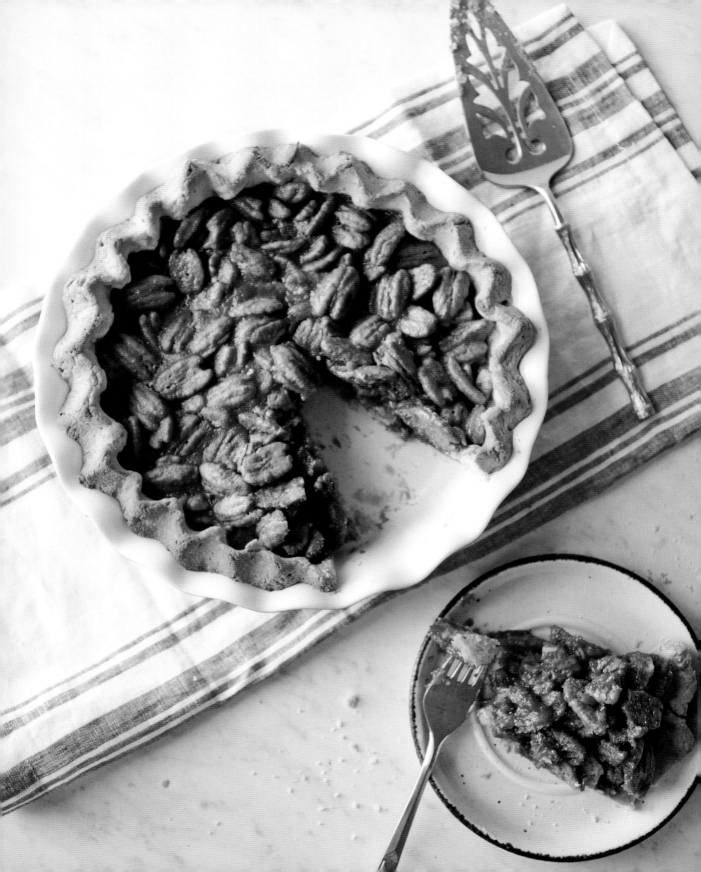

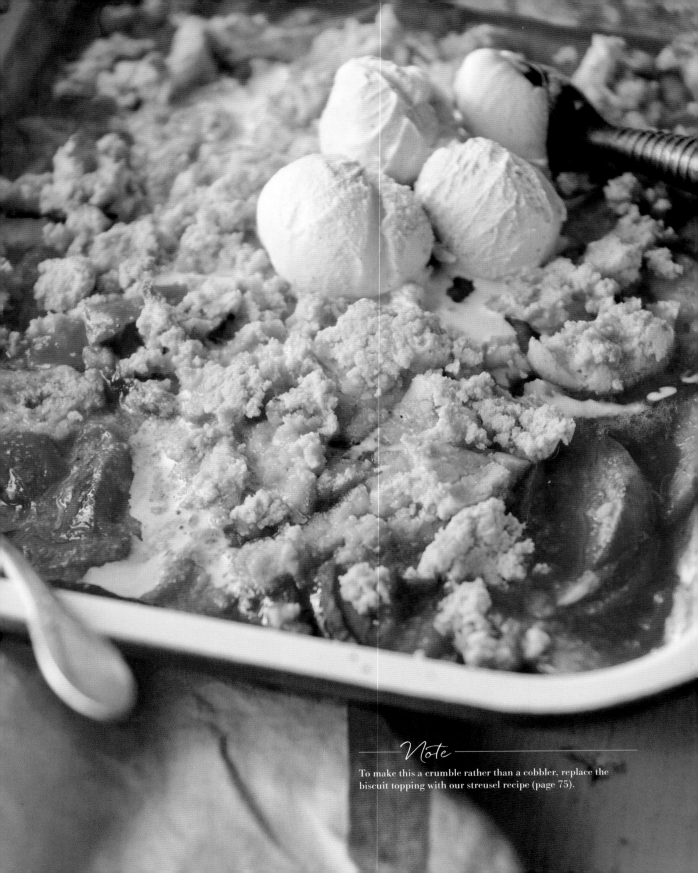

Note

To make this a crumble rather than a cobbler, replace the biscuit topping with our streusel recipe (page 75).

VANILLA BEAN PEACH COBBLER

When summer hits its peak, a peach cobbler feels necessary. It's the simplicity—fresh fruit, a golden brown crust, and of course some scoops of vanilla ice cream. In one bite it's warm and cold, creamy and crisp, sweet and tart. It's also ridiculously simple to put together and can be made for two dozen people almost as easily as for two. You just keep slicing peaches until your belly's full. Try it with any of your favorite fruits.

SERVES 8 TO 10

FOR THE FILLING

10 firm but ripe peaches, pitted and sliced (about 8 cups of sliced peaches)

¾ cup maple syrup

¼ cup fresh lemon juice

2 tablespoons arrowroot powder

¼ teaspoon Himalayan pink salt

2 teaspoons vanilla extract, or seeds from one vanila bean, scraped

FOR THE CRUST

1½ cups almond flour

¼ cup coconut flour

1 tablespoon baking powder

¼ teaspoon Himalayan pink salt

3 tablespoons maple syrup

¾ cup coconut yogurt, store-bought or homemade (page 40)

1 tablespoon vanilla extract

Creamy Dairy-Free Ice Cream (page 228) or Coconut Whipped Cream (page 30), for serving, optional

1. Preheat the oven to 400°F.

2. **MAKE THE FILLING:** In a large bowl, combine the peaches, maple syrup, lemon juice, arrowroot powder, salt, and vanilla. Stir well to combine. Scrape the mixture into a 9 × 13-inch baking dish. Bake for 15 to 20 minutes, until juicy and fragrant. Set aside while you make the cobbler crust. You can turn off the oven here, but you will need to preheat it again in about 45 minutes, while the dough finishes chilling (see step 4).

3. **MAKE THE CRUST:** In a medium bowl, whisk together the almond and coconut flours, baking powder, and salt. In a large bowl, combine the maple syrup, coconut yogurt, and vanilla. A little at a time, add the dry ingredients to the wet, stirring until a dough comes together.

4. Pat the dough into a ball. Press down until it forms a disk about 2 inches thick. Wrap in plastic and refrigerate for 1 hour. After about 45 minutes, preheat the oven again to 400°F.

5. Break off pieces of the dough and scatter all over the peaches, as evenly as you can. Return the cobbler to the oven and bake for 30 minutes, or until the topping is quite golden brown. Remove from the oven and let rest for at least 30 minutes so the peaches can set. Serve warm or at room temperature with ice cream or coconut whipped cream on the side.

TOASTED COCONUT CREAM PIE

This pie was inspired by Laurel's dear sister-in-law Corey, who bakes a coconut cream pie for every family gathering. She's blonde, always tan, and like most of Laurel's family, has some sand between her toes. The smooth coconut flavor in this pie is like a beach vacation in every bite. Because this pie has a custard filling, it will need to set for several hours. It's best started the day before you plan on serving it.

MAKES ONE 9-INCH PIE

FOR THE CRUST

2 tablespoons coconut oil, melted, plus more for greasing the pan

1½ cups almond flour

2 tablespoons unsweetened shredded coconut

1 teaspoon Himalayan pink salt

2 tablespoons maple syrup

FOR THE FILLING

One 13.5-ounce can full-fat coconut milk, refrigerated overnight

1 large egg

¼ cup arrowroot powder

3 tablespoons maple syrup

Pinch of Himalayan pink salt

½ cup unsweetened shredded coconut

1 teaspoon vanilla extract

Coconut Whipped Cream (page 30), for topping

Unsweetened flaked coconut, toasted (see Note), for topping

1. Preheat the oven to 350°F. Grease a 9-inch pie pan with coconut oil.

2. **MAKE THE CRUST:** In a medium bowl, whisk together the flour, coconut, and salt. In a separate medium bowl, combine the maple syrup and coconut oil. A little at a time, add the dry ingredients to the wet, stirring until a dough comes together. Gently press the dough into the pie pan and bake for 12 to 15 minutes, until golden brown. Allow to cool completely.

3. **MAKE THE FILLING:** Remove the solid coconut cream that has risen to the top of the coconut milk can and spoon it into a medium saucepan. Add the egg, arrowroot powder, maple syrup, and salt, and stir to fully blend; then bring to a simmer over medium-low heat, continuing to stir. Simmer until the mixture has thickened and the custard creates large, slow-to-pop bubbles, 15 to 20 minutes. Stir in the shredded coconut and vanilla and remove from the heat. Pour into a medium glass bowl, press plastic wrap onto the surface of the custard, and refrigerate, covered, for 30 minutes.

4. Pour the filling into the cooled crust and refrigerate for about 4 hours to set. Before serving, top with coconut whipped cream and toasted coconut flakes. Keep in the fridge for up to 4 days.

To properly toast coconut, it's all about timing. Spread dried coconut flakes onto a baking sheet and toast at 350°F for 10 to 15 minutes, or until the top layer of coconut is browned and the flakes smell fragrant. For a deeper toast, gently toss the coconut flakes on the baking sheet and toast for another 5 to 10 minutes, until evenly golden brown.

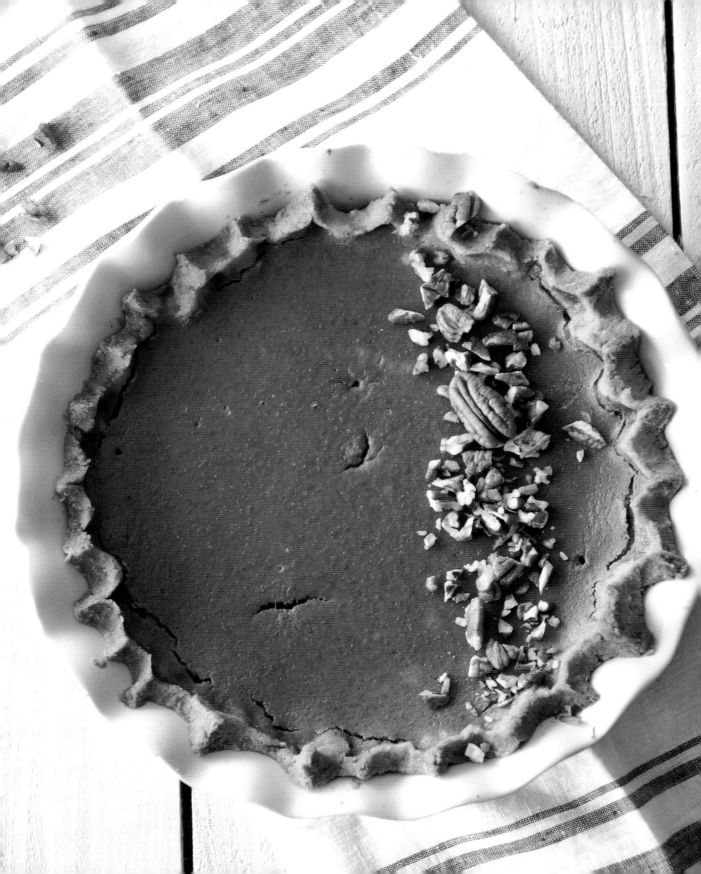

CLASSIC PUMPKIN PIE

Cinnamon is the spice that Claire teases Laurel about the most. Laurel will put a tablespoon in a recipe without even blinking, she loves it so much—that's a lot of cinnamon! Other than its lovely, warm flavor, it's also an impressive antioxidant. And in this creamy pumpkin pie, we use plenty of it, along with other classic spices for a full-bodied holiday flavor.

MAKES ONE 9-INCH PIE

FOR THE CRUST

¼ cup coconut oil, solid

2½ cups almond flour

1 cup arrowroot powder

Pinch of Himalayan pink salt

¼ cup maple syrup

1 large egg

Coconut oil, for greasing the pan

FOR THE FILLING

1¾ cups pumpkin puree

3 large eggs

½ cup full-fat coconut milk or almond milk

⅓ cup maple syrup

1 teaspoon vanilla extract

1 tablespoon ground cinnamon

½ teaspoon grated nutmeg

½ teaspoon ground ginger

¼ teaspoon ground cloves

Pinch of Himalayan pink salt

Coconut Whipped Cream (page 30), for serving

1. **MAKE THE CRUST:** Combine the coconut oil, flour, arrowroot powder, and salt in a large bowl and mix with a pastry blender or your fingertips until a dough comes together. Stir in the maple syrup and egg. Gently shape the dough into a ball, cover with plastic wrap, and chill in the fridge for about an hour.

2. Preheat the oven to 350°F. Grease a 9-inch pie pan with coconut oil.

3. **MAKE THE FILLING:** In a large bowl using a hand mixer, beat together the pumpkin puree and eggs. Add the milk, maple syrup, vanilla, cinnamon, nutmeg, ginger, cloves, and salt and blend until smooth.

4. Remove the dough from the fridge and allow to thaw, about 10 minutes. Roll the dough about ¼ inch thick. Place it in the pie pan and trim any excess. Pour the filling into the crust.

5. Bake for 30 minutes, until the filling is set at the edges but jiggly in the center. The piecrust can easily get overcooked, so for this recipe we like to shield the edges with strips of aluminum foil. After 30 minutes, remove the foil strips and continue to bake until the center of the pie just barely jiggles, 15 to 20 more minutes. Cool to room temperature before serving with lots of coconut whipped cream. Refrigerate for up to 4 days.

CREAMY DAIRY-FREE CHEESECAKE

Creamy and rich with a bit of tartness, cheesecake is a delicious canvas for other flavors, like fresh fruit, strawberry sauce, a drizzle of vegan caramel, or your favorite spices. This is our classic, no-nonsense recipe—feel free to make it your own.

MAKES ONE 9-INCH CHEESECAKE

FOR THE CRUST

3 tablespoons coconut oil, melted, plus more for greasing the pan

6 Graham Crackers (page 104)

Pinch of Himalayan pink salt

2 tablespoons maple syrup

FOR THE FILLING

2¾ cups coconut yogurt, store-bought or homemade (page 40)

½ cup maple syrup

¼ cup date paste, store-bought or homemade (page 42)

5 large eggs

¼ cup arrowroot powder

1 tablespoon fresh lemon juice

1 teaspoon vanilla extract

Coconut Sour Cream (recipe follows), for serving

1. Preheat the oven to 325°F. Generously grease a 9-inch springform pan with coconut oil.

2. **MAKE THE CRUST:** Pulse together the graham crackers, coconut oil, salt, and maple syrup in a food processor until the mixture forms a ball. Lightly press the dough into the prepared pan.

3. **MAKE THE FILLING:** In a food processor, pulse together the coconut yogurt, maple syrup, and date paste until combined. Transfer the mixture to a medium bowl and whisk in the eggs, arrowroot powder, lemon juice, and vanilla until smooth.

4. Pour the filling into the crust and bake for 45 to 55 minutes, until set on the edges and barely jiggly in the center. Allow the cake to cool completely, then top with the coconut sour cream. Refrigerate for up to 3 days.

—— *Note* ——

Cracks in cheesecake can be frustrating. To prevent them, be careful not to overbeat the filling, always grease the sides of the pan, keep the oven temperature low (300°F to 325°F is best), and cool the cheesecake slowly—never put it straight into the fridge.

Coconut Sour Cream

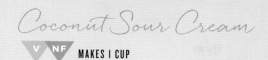

V NF MAKES 1 CUP

One 13.5-ounce can full-fat coconut milk, refrigerated overnight

1 tablespoon coconut yogurt, store-bought or homemade (page 40)

1 teaspoon lemon juice

1 tablespoon maple syrup

½ teaspoon vanilla extract

1. Spoon the solid coconut cream that has risen to the top of the can into the bowl of a stand mixer fitted with the whisk attachment. Beat the coconut cream on high speed until it begins to thicken and peaks form.

2. Using a rubber spatula, slowly fold in the coconut yogurt, lemon juice, maple syrup, and vanilla. Transfer the sour cream to a metal bowl and refrigerate, covered, until ready to use, for up to 5 days.

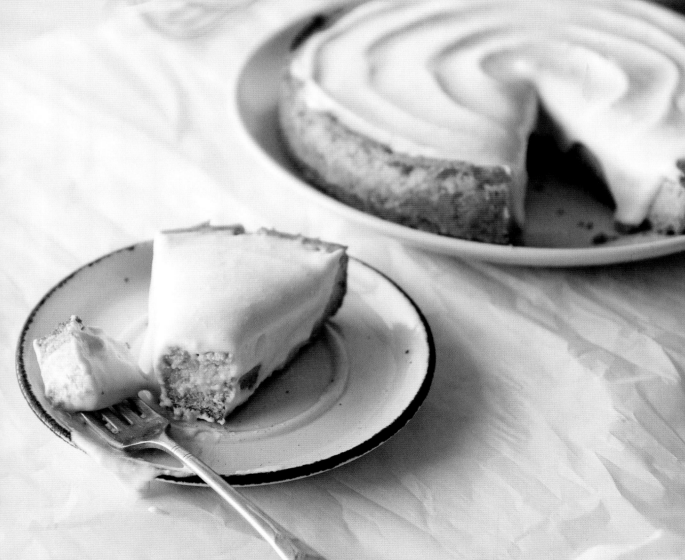

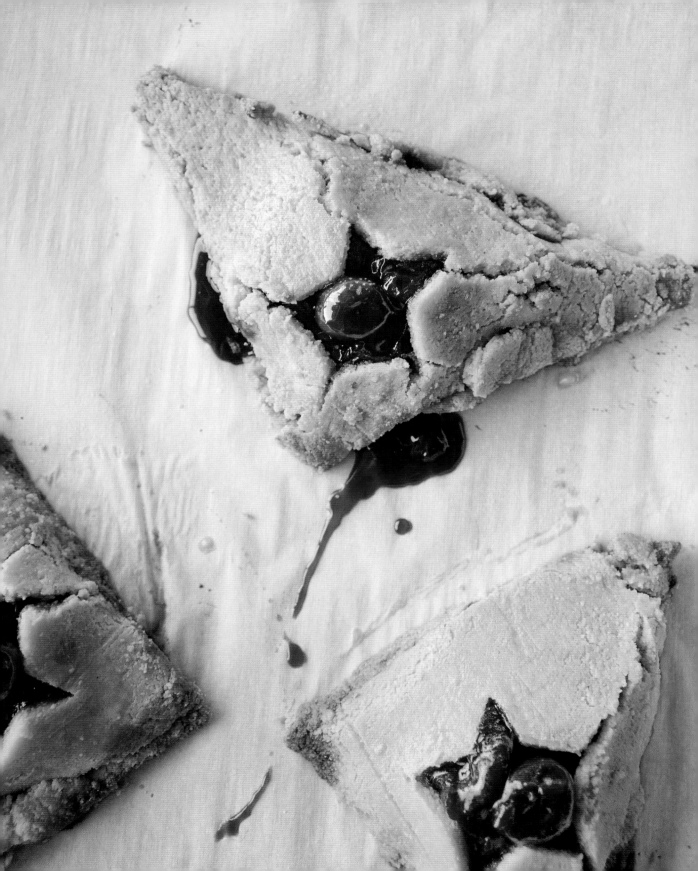

SALTY'S CHERRY HAND PIES

Cherry pie is Laurel's dad's all-time favorite, and that's why she named our version after him, who's lovingly called "Salty" by her mom—though we all agree he is sweet as can be. (That's another story for another time!) These little hand pies are perfect for an end-of-summer grill-out, and can be made with any fruit filling you like.

MAKES 6 HAND PIES

FOR THE CRUST

2½ cups almond flour

1 cup arrowroot powder

¼ cup maple syrup

1 large egg

Pinch of Himalayan pink salt

¼ cup coconut oil, solid

FOR THE FILLING

4 cups frozen or fresh cherries, pitted

½ cup maple syrup

Juice of 1 lemon

1 tablespoon arrowroot powder

1 large egg, beaten

1. Preheat the oven to 350°F. Line a baking sheet with parchment paper.

2. **MAKE THE CRUST:** Combine the flour, arrowroot powder, maple syrup, egg, salt, and coconut oil in a large bowl and mix with a pastry blender or your fingertips until a dough comes together. Gently shape the dough into a ball, cover with plastic wrap, and chill in the freezer for about an hour.

3. Place the dough between two pieces of parchment paper and roll it out ¼ inch thick. Remove the top piece of parchment and, using a paring knife, cut the dough into six 5 × 5-inch squares. Then, use a 1- to 2-inch star-shaped cookie cutter to cut out a star from each square. The goal is that when you fold the square over on the diagonal, the star shape will be in the center of the turnover. Place the squares of dough on the prepared baking sheet with a spatula. Chill in the refrigerator while you prepare the filling.

4. **MAKE THE FILLING:** In a medium saucepan over medium heat, combine the cherries, maple syrup, and lemon juice. Cook for about 10 minutes, until the mixture begins to boil; then remove the pan from the heat and stir in the arrowroot powder.

5. Place 2 heaping tablespoons of the cherry mixture in the center of each dough square. Fold one corner of the dough up over the cherry mixture to form a triangle, and seal the edges by crimping with fork tines. Don't worry if there are breaks along the folded edge, just pinch the dough down with your fingertips to reseal.

6. Brush some egg over each hand pie. Bake for about 30 minutes, until golden brown and any cherry liquid dripping out appears thick. Serve immediately or refrigerate for up to 2 days. Rewarm before serving.

SALTED LEMON MERINGUE PIE

Lemon meringue pie is a classic. Being lemon-obsessed girls (Laurel actually eats lemons like apples while Claire looks on, completely mystified), we agree this pie is one of our personal favorites. The touch of salt brings out the sweetness and bright flavors in this pie, while the meringue floats on top like a cloud. The filling will need to set in the refrigerator, so be sure to plan ahead.

MAKES ONE 9-INCH PIE

FOR THE CRUST

2 tablespoons coconut oil, solid, plus more for greasing the pan

2 cups almond flour

1 tablespoon maple syrup

½ teaspoon Himalayan pink salt

FOR THE FILLING

½ cup maple syrup

¼ cup arrowroot powder

6 large egg yolks

Grated zest and juice of 4 lemons

1½ tablespoons coconut oil, solid

FOR THE MERINGUE

6 large egg whites, at room temperature

1 teaspoon cream of tartar

Pinch of Himalayan pink salt

3 tablespoons maple syrup

1. Preheat the oven to 350°F. Grease a 9-inch pie pan with coconut oil.

2. **MAKE THE CRUST:** Combine the coconut oil, flour, maple syrup, and salt in a medium bowl and mix with a pastry blender until a dough comes together. It will be a bit sandy in texture, not a sticky dough. Lightly press the dough into the pie pan and bake for about 15 to 20 minutes, until light golden brown.

3. **MAKE THE FILLING:** In a medium saucepan over medium heat, stir together the maple syrup and arrowroot powder. Add 1 cup water and bring the mixture to a simmer. To prevent the eggs from curdling, temper them first: In a small bowl, add a small amount of the maple mixture to the beaten egg yolks in a constant drizzle, stirring to combine. Once you've added about one-fourth of the maple mixture, add the egg mixture slowly back to the saucepan of the maple mixture, whisking constantly to combine. Mix in the lemon zest and juice, and return the mixture to a simmer. Cook for 3 to 5 minutes, until thickened, then remove the mixture from the heat and stir in the coconut oil.

4. Pour the filling into the piecrust and place in the refrigerator to set for at least 4 hours, then prepare the topping.

5. **MAKE THE MERINGUE:** In the bowl of a stand mixer fitted with the whisk attachment, combine the egg whites, cream of tartar, and salt. Beat on high for 3 minutes until stiff peaks form, then slowly add the maple syrup.

6. Dollop the meringue all over the chilled filling to the edge of the crust. Toast with a butane torch or carefully broil, checking it every 30 seconds. Serve immediately or refrigerate for up to a day before serving.

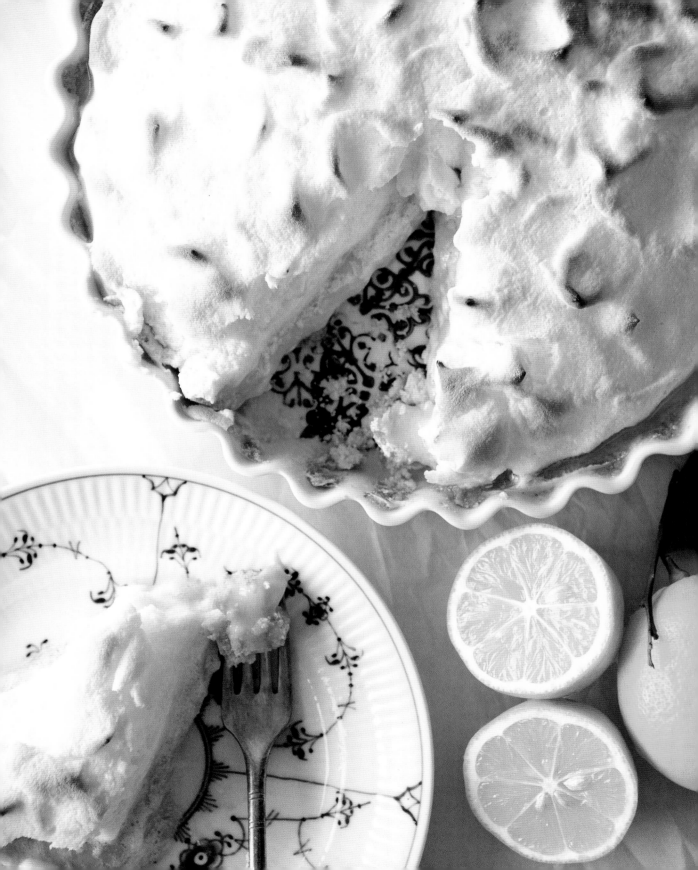

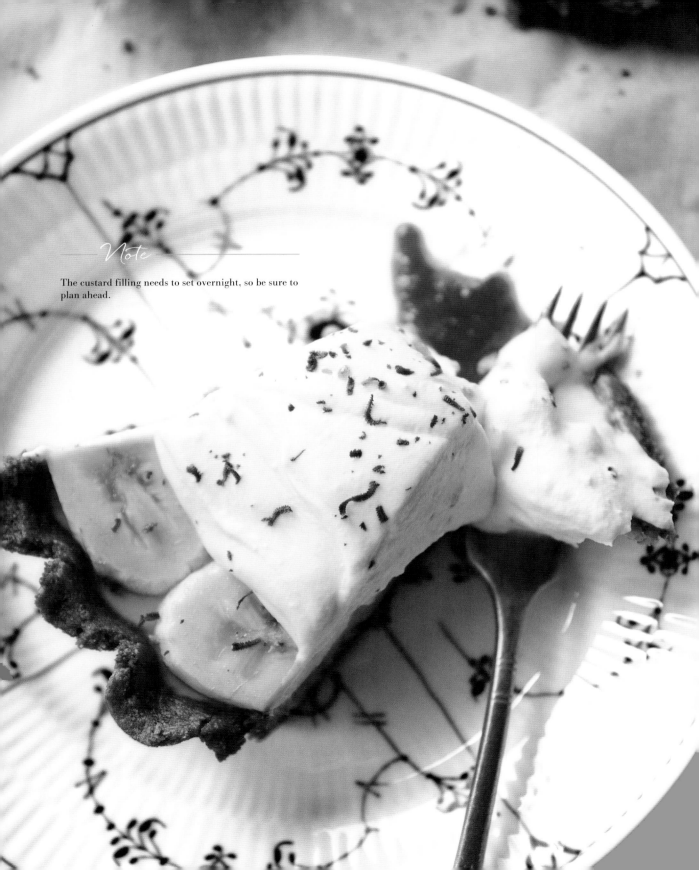

Note

The custard filling needs to set overnight, so be sure to plan ahead.

CARAMEL CHOCOLATE BANANA CREAM PIE

We started with our favorite banana cream pie, and then kept adding more delicious ingredients to it—chocolate in the crust, a swirl of caramel, grated chocolate on top. And we like this pie even better with the slightest dusting of salt, which really brings out the caramel notes. It's delicious served sliced, but also wonderful as banana pudding served in a bowl.

MAKES ONE 9-INCH PIE

FOR THE CRUST

¼ cup coconut oil, solid, plus more for greasing the pan

2½ cups almond flour

3 tablespoons 100% unsweetened cacao powder

¾ cup plus 1 tablespoon arrowroot powder

¼ cup maple syrup

1 large egg

Pinch of Himalayan pink salt

¾ cup Vegan Caramel (page 40)

FOR THE FILLING

3 cups full-fat coconut milk

1 tablespoon gelatin powder

3 large egg yolks

¼ cup maple syrup

2 teaspoons vanilla extract

¼ teaspoon Himalayan pink salt

2 bananas, sliced

Coconut Whipped Cream (page 30), for serving

100% cacao unsweetened baking chocolate shavings, for garnish

1. Preheat the oven to 350°F. Grease a 9-inch pie pan with coconut oil.

2. **MAKE THE CRUST:** Combine the flour, cacao powder, arrowroot powder, maple syrup, coconut oil, egg, and salt in a large bowl and mix with a pastry blender until a dough forms. Gently shape into a ball, cover with plastic wrap, and refrigerate for 30 minutes.

3. Roll out the dough about ¼ inch thick. Place in the pie pan, trim any excess, and bake for about 10 minutes, until set. Allow to cool, then pour ½ cup of the caramel into the crust and smooth into an even layer. Chill in the refrigerator for at least 30 minutes.

4. **MAKE THE FILLING:** Pour the coconut milk into a medium saucepan and sprinkle the gelatin on top. Allow the gelatin to soften for about 5 minutes. In a medium bowl, whisk together the egg yolks, maple syrup, and vanilla.

5. Cook the coconut milk and gelatin, whisking, over low heat until smooth and warm, about 5 minutes. Add a cup of the warm coconut milk mixture to the egg yolk mixture, stirring constantly. Pour the entire yolk mixture into the saucepan and mix well. Add the salt and, whisking constantly, simmer for about 10 minutes, until the filling begins to thicken. The custard is ready when it coats the back of a spoon. Allow to cool for 1 hour, then pour it into the cooled crust and refrigerate for 8 hours or overnight.

6. To serve, arrange banana slices over the chilled custard and top with the coconut whipped cream, the remaining ¼ cup caramel, and shaved cacao.

LAUREL'S BAKLAVA PIE

Any good Grecian girl loves her baklava! Laurel created this recipe in honor of her favorite traditional Greek treat, which was central to our early years of friendship. The first thing we baked together was an orange- and cinnamon-infused baklava. We wanted to be sure this pie was just as flavorful as that was—and it is. Disclaimer: This pie smells sinfully good while baking, and tastes even better as you take your first bite.

MAKES ONE 9-INCH PIE

FOR THE CRUST

2 tablespoons coconut oil, solid, plus more for greasing the pan

2 cups almond flour

1 tablespoon ground cinnamon

1 teaspoon Himalayan pink salt

2 tablespoons maple syrup

FOR THE FILLING

¼ cup date paste, store-bought or homemade (page 42)

1 cup honey

Rind from 1 orange

3 cinnamon sticks

3 large eggs

¼ cup coconut oil, solid

1 tablespoon vanilla extract

1 tablespoon ground cinnamon

1 teaspoon Himalayan pink salt

3 cups walnuts, coarsely ground

1. Preheat the oven to 350°F. Line a 9-inch pie pan with a parchment paper round and grease the pan with coconut oil.

2. **MAKE THE CRUST:** In a medium bowl, stir together the coconut oil, flour, cinnamon, salt, and maple syrup until a dough forms. Lightly press the dough into the pie pan. Set aside while you prepare the filling.

3. **MAKE THE FILLING:** Pulse together the date paste and honey in a blender or food processor until the mixture becomes liquid. Transfer the mixture to a medium saucepan set over medium heat and add the orange rind and cinnamon sticks. Simmer for 10 minutes, until the syrup is very aromatic and slightly thickened. Remove the orange rind and cinnamon sticks, and allow the mixture to cool completely.

4. In a medium bowl, beat the eggs, coconut oil, vanilla, cinnamon, and salt until smooth. Gradually add the syrup and walnuts, stirring to combine well. Pour the filling into the crust and bake for 40 to 50 minutes, until set. Serve warm or at room temperature, or refrigerate for up to 5 days.

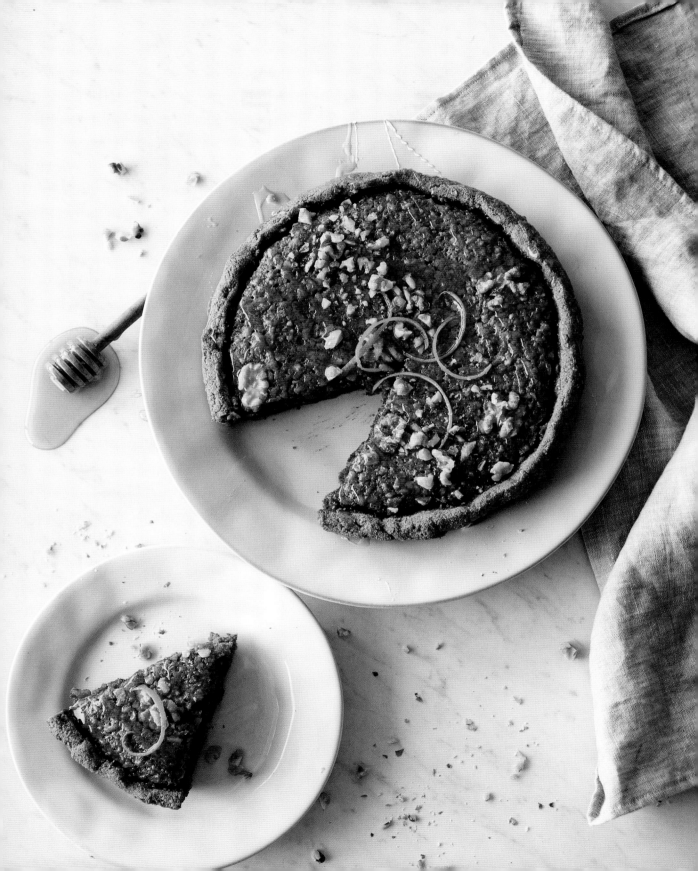

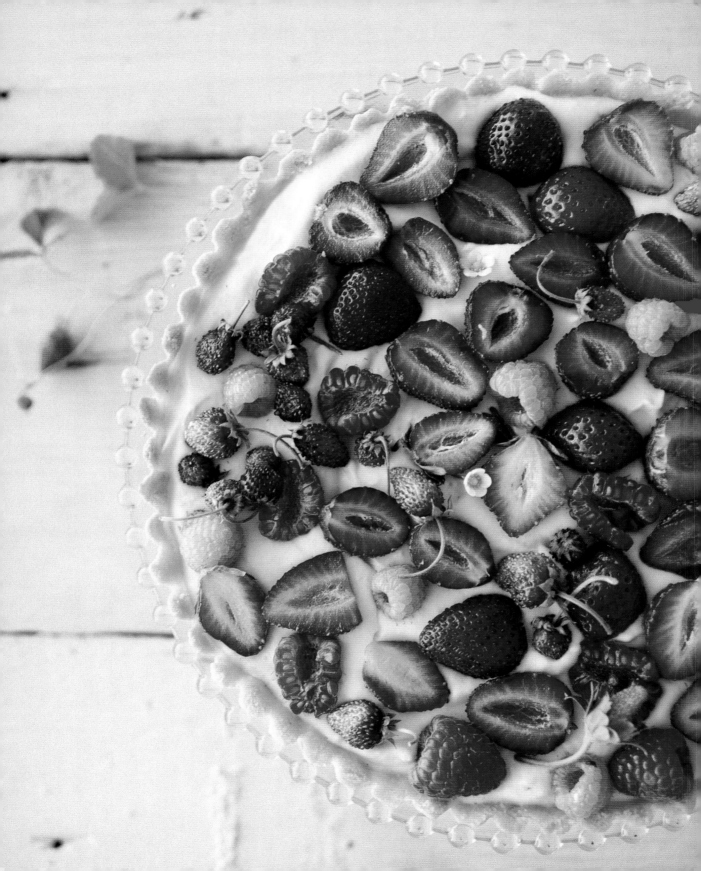

SUMMER STRAWBERRY TART

Delicate coconut whipped cream topped with beautiful fresh berries—what more could you ask for? We wanted to create a pie that highlights summer's bountiful produce. This pie shows the simplistic beauty we always strive for at Sweet Laurel, letting nature take its turn and showing off its beautiful accents. Inspired by a tart Claire enjoyed on her springtime honeymoon in Rome, this is our favorite pie to enjoy on long summer evenings, when a high-maintenance dessert is the last thing on your mind. Try it with any peak-season summer fruit. Ripe cherries, small French plums . . . anything from the farmer's market would be a wonderful addition to this recipe.

MAKES ONE 9-INCH TART

2 tablespoons coconut oil, solid, plus more for greasing the pan

2 cups plus 2 tablespoons almond flour

¼ teaspoon Himalayan pink salt

1 tablespoon maple syrup

1 large egg

2 cups Coconut Whipped Cream (page 30)

4 cups strawberries, mix of whole, halved, and sliced

1. Preheat the oven to 350°F. Generously grease a 9-inch tart pan with coconut oil.

2. In a food processor fitted with the chopping blade, pulse the flour and salt until combined. Add the coconut oil, maple syrup, and egg and blend until the mixture forms a ball. Lightly press the dough into the tart pan and bake for 10 to 12 minutes, until light golden brown.

3. Remove the crust from the oven and allow to cool completely. Fill the crust with coconut whipped cream and top with strawberries. Slice and serve. This is best the same day it is made, but the crust can be made up to a week ahead of time and stored, well wrapped, in the fridge.

PEAR FRANGIPANE GALETTE

Few things seem more effortless than a rustic galette, a hand-made tart. It has this air of, "Oh, this? I just whipped it up with the pears from my garden." Of course, most of us aren't living in such a hostess fantasy, but serving up this simple galette can help us feel one step closer to it. We love this recipe with fall pears atop a pillow of sweet frangipane. It's not too sweet, and makes a lovely, simple end to a casual dinner.

MAKES ONE 8-INCH TART

FOR THE FILLING

2 to 3 pears, peeled, halved, and cored

1 teaspoon fresh lemon juice

1 tablespoon ground cinnamon

1 cup blanched almonds

¼ cup coconut oil, melted

3 tablespoons date paste, store-bought or homemade (page 42)

2 large eggs

½ teaspoon vanilla extract

¼ teaspoon Himalayan pink salt

FOR THE CRUST

2 cups almond flour

½ cup arrowroot powder

¼ teaspoon Himalayan pink salt

¼ cup coconut oil, solid

3 tablespoons maple syrup

1 teaspoon vanilla extract

Two-Ingredient Ice Cream (page 226) or Creamy Dairy-Free Ice Cream (page 228), for serving

1. Preheat the oven to 350°F. Line a baking sheet with parchment paper.

2. **MAKE THE FILLING:** Slice the pear halves into 8 pieces each, then place the slices in a medium bowl and toss together with the lemon juice and cinnamon.

3. Pulse the almonds, coconut oil, and date paste in a food processor until you have a cohesive paste. Add the eggs, vanilla, and salt and pulse again until smooth.

4. **MAKE THE CRUST:** In a medium bowl, whisk together the flour, arrowroot powder, and salt. In a separate medium bowl, combine the coconut oil, maple syrup, and vanilla. A little at a time, add the dry ingredients to the wet, stirring until a dough comes together.

5. Place the dough between two pieces of parchment paper and roll it about 10 inches wide and ⅛ inch thick. Remove the top piece of paper and spoon the date filling into the center, leaving a 1-inch border all around. Arrange the pears on top of the date filling in a windmill pattern. Fold the dough edges up over the filling, pressing down to secure. Bake for 25 to 30 minutes, until the pears are tender and the crust is golden brown. Serve immediately with a scoop of ice cream or refrigerate for up to 2 days; rewarm before serving.

— Note —

You can try this recipe with practically any fruit, but we especially love it with summer stone fruits.

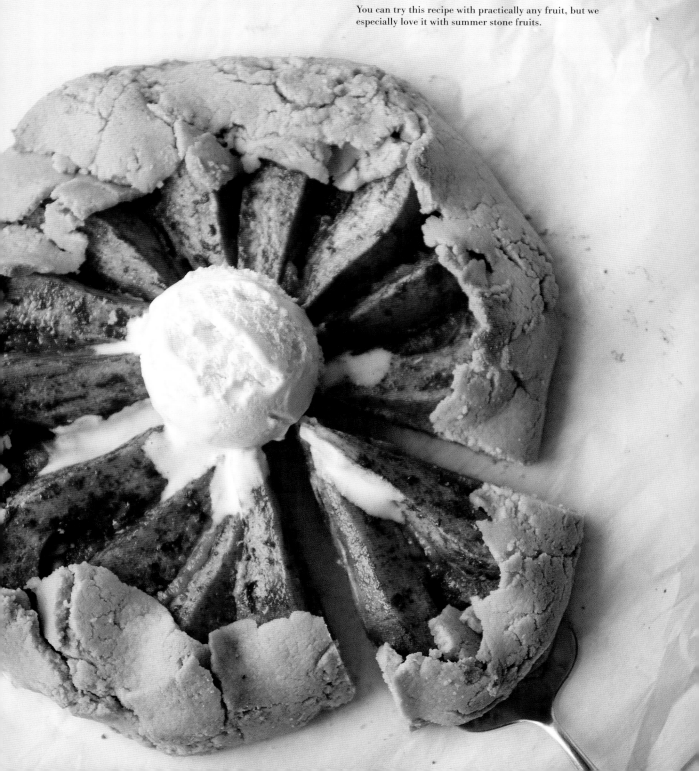

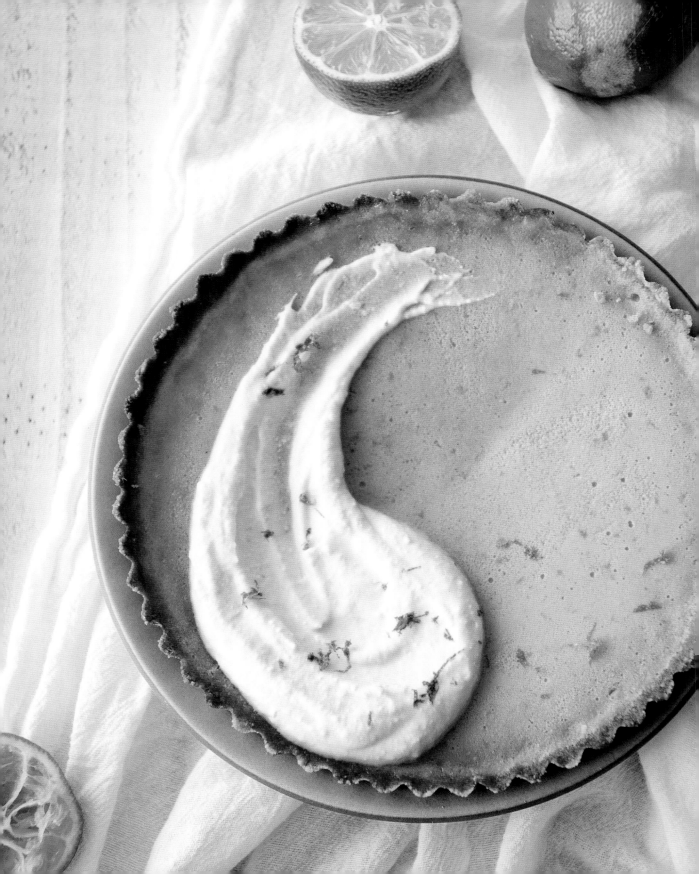

ZESTY LIME PIE
with COCONUT CRUST

This lime filling pairs especially well with the coconut crust, giving you bright, tropical flavors in every bite. This same concept works beautifully with any citrus you prefer—or even passion fruit if you can find it. The custard filling needs to set overnight, so be sure to plan ahead.

MAKES ONE 9-INCH PIE

FOR THE CRUST

2 tablespoons coconut oil, melted, plus more for greasing the pan

1½ cups almond flour

2 tablespoons unsweetened shredded coconut

½ teaspoon Himalayan pink salt

2 tablespoons maple syrup

FOR THE FILLING

3 large eggs

½ cup maple syrup

½ cup full-fat coconut milk

½ cup fresh lime juice, plus grated zest of 1 lime

2 tablespoons arrowroot powder

Lime Coconut Whipped Cream (page 31), for serving

1. Preheat the oven to 350°F. Generously grease a 9-inch pie or tart pan with coconut oil.

2. **MAKE THE CRUST:** In a medium bowl, whisk together the flour, shredded coconut, and salt. In a separate medium bowl, combine the maple syrup and coconut oil. A little at a time, add the dry ingredients to the wet, stirring until a dough comes together. Gently press the dough into the pie pan and bake for about 12 minutes, until golden brown. Allow to cool completely.

3. **MAKE THE FILLING:** In a large bowl, whisk together the eggs and maple syrup. Add the coconut milk, lime juice and zest, and arrowroot powder and whisk until completely smooth.

4. The piecrust can easily get overcooked, so for this recipe we like to shield the edges with strips of aluminum foil. Reduce the oven temperature to 325°F. Pour the filling into the crust. Bake for 30 to 40 minutes, until the pie is set at the edges and barely jiggly in the middle. Refrigerate for at least 8 hours. Top with lime coconut whipped cream before serving. The pie will keep in the fridge for up to 2 days.

NO-BAKE CHEESECAKE
with SIMMERED APRICOTS AND PISTACHIO CRUST

A vegan "cheesecake" with dried fruit and a nut crust doesn't sound particularly sexy, but when the cheesecake is decadent and creamy, the dried fruit is rendered soft and syrupy, and the nut crust is dotted with gem-like pistachios, it's hard to pass up a slice. This recipe is our favorite "break open in case of emergencies" dessert, because it can be made weeks ahead of time and will delight even the pickiest eaters. The best part is the versatility. The crust can be made with any nut; the filling can have fruit zest, spices, or cacao added; and the syrupy topping can be made with any dried fruit—cherries, figs, prunes, you name it.

SERVES 16 TO 20

FOR THE CRUST

2 cups coarsely ground pistachios

¼ teaspoon Himalayan pink salt

1 tablespoon coconut oil, melted

¼ cup date paste, store-bought or homemade (page 42)

FOR THE FILLING

3 cups raw cashews, soaked overnight in water

⅔ cup fresh lemon juice

⅔ cup coconut oil, melted

1¼ cups coconut cream (about two 13.5-ounce cans of full-fat coconut milk)

1 cup maple syrup

1 tablespoon vanilla extract

¼ teaspoon Himalayan pink salt

1. Line a 9 × 13-inch baking dish with parchment paper, letting the paper hang over the sides for easy removal.

2. **MAKE THE CRUST:** Combine the pistachios, salt, coconut oil, and date paste in a medium bowl and stir into a pliable dough. Firmly press the mixture into the lined dish. Set aside.

3. **MAKE THE FILLING:** Drain the cashews, then place in a blender along with the lemon juice, coconut oil, coconut cream, maple syrup, vanilla, and salt. Blend until very smooth and velvety. Be sure there aren't any chunks of cashew. If the mixture proves too thick to puree smoothly, just add a little of the leftover coconut liquid from the can, a tablespoon at a time.

4. Pour the mixture over the crust. Lift up the pan and tap it on the counter a few times to release any air bubbles, then cover with plastic wrap and freeze until set—4 to 6 hours. You can then hold it in the fridge until you're ready to finish.

FOR THE TOPPING

1½ pounds pitted dried apricots (or any dried fruit) (about 50 apricots)

1 cup maple syrup

2 cinnamon sticks

Zest of 1 orange

2 cups fresh orange juice

5. **MAKE THE TOPPING:** In a medium saucepan over medium-high heat, combine the apricots, maple syrup, cinnamon sticks, orange zest, orange juice, and 1 cup water. Bring to a boil, then reduce to a simmer and cook for 45 to 50 minutes, until the liquid has turned to syrup and the fruit is completely tender. You should be able to cut and bite through it without much effort. If it needs more time, cook it for another 5 minutes and test it again.

6. Strain the fruit into a bowl to cool completely, about 1 hour (or less in the fridge). Discard the cinnamon sticks and orange zest. In the same saucepan, reduce the remaining syrup over medium heat for another 15 minutes, or until it becomes thick and syrupy. Set aside to cool completely. We usually pour the syrup back over the fruit and hold it in the fridge until we're ready to use it.

7. To serve, take the cheesecake from the fridge and spoon the fruit on top, covering the whole cheesecake. Drizzle with syrup. If you're making this ahead of time, keep the cheesecake and fruit with syrup separate until serving. The cheesecake can be made a week beforehand if kept in the freezer, and the fruit 2 weeks ahead if refrigerated in a sealed container.

—— *Notes* ——

We like to keep our ingredients as clean as possible, so any dried fruit we work with is sulfite-free. This means the fruit tends to have a ruddier, browner hue, but it still has the same fabulous flavor.

The topping can be made weeks ahead of time if refrigerated in a sealed container, and is delicious as a dessert or porridge topping. It can also be turned into a delicious jam by simply pureeing the fruit and syrup.

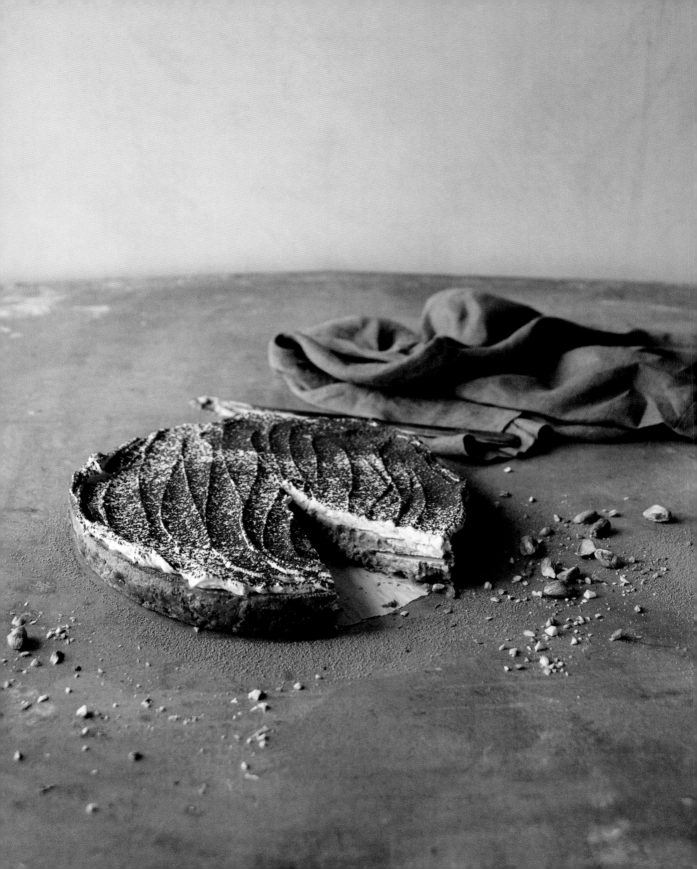

MATCHA CUSTARD PIE
with PISTACHIO CRUST

We knew a creamy custard pie would contrast beautifully against the fresh, earthy, and slightly bitter notes of our favorite powdered green tea. With pistachios in the crust, every bite of this dessert has a pop of gorgeous green. For the most vibrant pie, be sure to use fresh matcha. The pie needs to set overnight, so be sure to plan ahead.

MAKES ONE 9-INCH PIE

FOR THE CRUST

2 tablespoons coconut oil, melted, plus more for greasing the pan

2 cups coarsely ground pistachios

¼ teaspoon Himalayan pink salt

1 tablespoon maple syrup

1 large egg

FOR THE FILLING

One 13.5-ounce can full-fat coconut milk

2 tablespoons honey

4 large eggs

2 tablespoons matcha powder, sifted, plus more for serving

1. Preheat the oven to 325°F. Grease a 9-inch springform pan with coconut oil and securely cover the exterior of the pan with foil to cover the bottom and up the sides.

2. **MAKE THE CRUST:** In a medium bowl, stir until well combined the coconut oil, pistachios, salt, maple syrup, and egg. Firmly press the mixture into the base of the springform pan and set aside.

3. **MAKE THE FILLING:** In a teakettle or a medium pot, bring 2 to 3 cups of water to a boil over high heat (you'll want this for the water bath). In a separate medium pot, bring the coconut milk and honey to a simmer over medium heat, simmering for 5 minutes. Remove from the heat.

4. In a medium bowl, whisk together the eggs and matcha. To prevent the eggs from curdling, temper them first. In a small bowl, add a small amount of the coconut mixture to the eggs and matcha in a constant drizzle, stirring to combine. Once you've added about one-fourth of the coconut mixture, add the egg and matcha mixture slowly back into the saucepan of the coconut mixture, whisking constantly to combine.

5. Place the springform pan in a baking dish at least 2 inches deep, and pour in hot water so it covers the bottom inch of the springform. Pour the filling into the springform and bake for 45 to 60 minutes, until the filling is set around the edges but jiggles a bit in the center. Refrigerate the pie for 8 hours or overnight to finish setting. Serve with a heavy dusting of matcha on top. The pie will keep in the fridge for up to 3 days.

CLASSIC SWEET POTATO MAPLE PIE

Sliceable velvet, that's what this pie is. Delicately spiced and beautifully hued, this unexpected alternative to pumpkin pie is one of our Thanksgiving favorites. It's subtler than typical holiday desserts and perfectly delicious.

MAKES ONE 9-INCH PIE

FOR THE CRUST

2½ cups almond flour

1 cup arrowroot powder

Pinch of Himalayan pink salt

¼ cup coconut oil, solid, plus more for greasing the parchment

¼ cup maple syrup

1 large egg

FOR THE FILLING

1 pound sweet potato

⅓ cup coconut oil, solid

½ cup maple syrup

½ cup full-fat coconut milk

2 large eggs

½ teaspoon grated nutmeg

½ teaspoon ground cinnamon

1 teaspoon vanilla extract

1. **MAKE THE CRUST:** In a medium bowl, whisk together the flour, arrowroot powder, and salt. Cut the coconut oil into the dry ingredients with a pastry blender or your fingertips until a dough comes together. It will look like wet sand, and the fats should be pea-size. Stir in the maple syrup and egg until fully incorporated. Gently shape the dough into a ball, cover with plastic wrap, press into a disk, and chill in the freezer for about 2 hours.

2. Preheat the oven to 350°F. Grease a 9-inch pie pan with coconut oil.

3. Place the chilled pie dough between two large pieces of parchment, sprinkling the top of the dough with a little arrowroot to prevent sticking. Roll it into a circle about ⅛ inch thick and 11 inches wide. Roll the dough up around the rolling pin—don't worry if it cracks a little—then roll it across the pie pan and gently press the dough in place. Press any cracks together. Trim the edges and decorate however you prefer, though we usually keep it very simple, with a basic smooth or fluted edge. Prick the pie dough with a fork all over, to prevent it from rising in the oven. Pop the crust back in the fridge for 10 minutes to chill.

4. Bake the piecrust for 15 minutes, until firm but not golden brown. Let cool while you work on the filling.

5. **MAKE THE FILLING:** Boil the whole sweet potato in a medium pot of water over medium heat for 40 to 50 minutes, or until tender. (You can also microwave the potato for 10 to 15 minutes.) Run cold water over the sweet potato and remove the skin.

Note

For the best results and easiest handling, keep the pie dough thoroughly chilled. As you're rolling or shaping it, it should feel cold to the touch. If not, just pop the dough back in the fridge for 10 minutes to rechill.

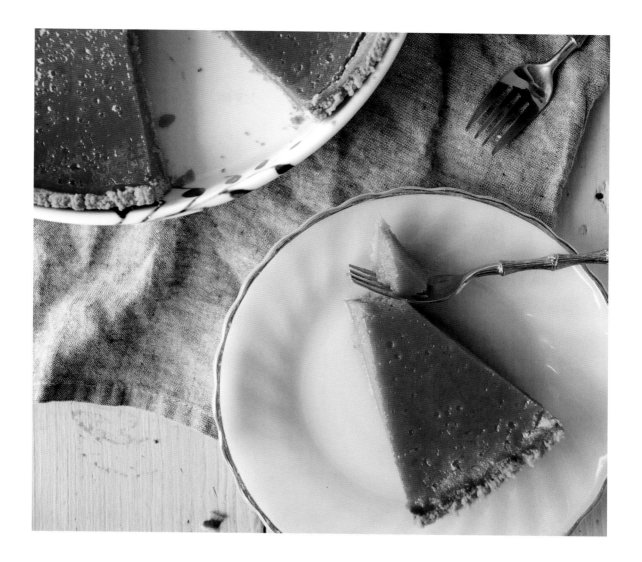

6. Put the sweet potato in a medium bowl and break it into chunks. Add the coconut oil and beat until smooth with an electric mixer. Mix in the maple syrup, coconut milk, eggs, nutmeg, cinnamon, and vanilla. Continue beating on medium speed until the mixture is smooth. Pour the mixture into the prebaked piecrust.

7. Bake for 55 to 60 minutes, or until a knife inserted into the center comes out clean. Cool completely before serving.

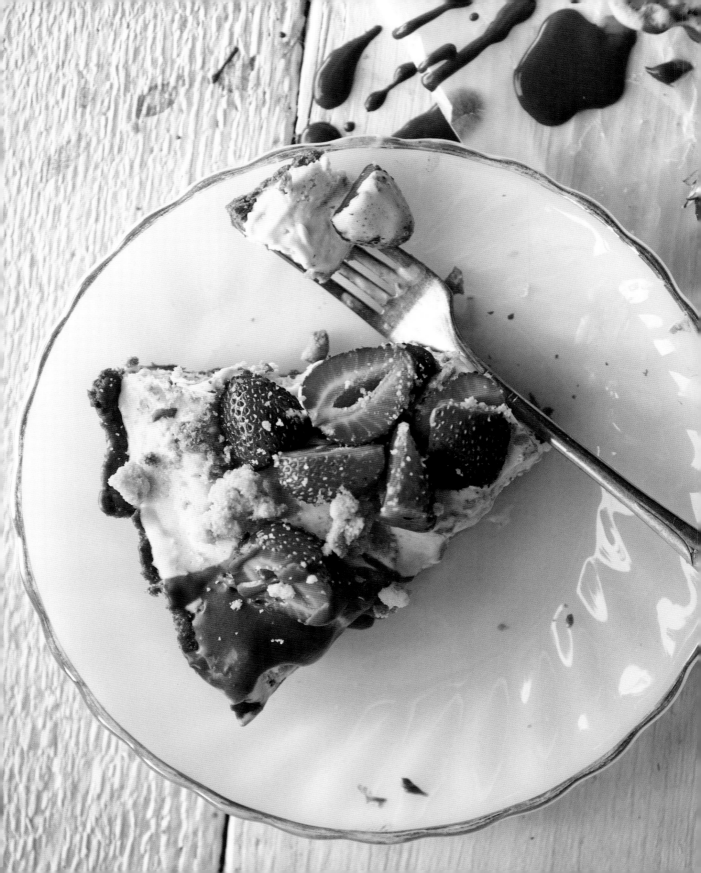

CHOCOLATE-STRAWBERRY MELT-AWAY PIE

Melt-away pie has such a romantic sound to it. Like warm summer nights giving way to fall, it has an ephemeral quality. But in truth, it's simply an ice cream pie, and it couldn't be easier to put together. The base is a piecrust with ice cream filling, and the toppings can be whatever sundae fantasy you feel like that day. We love the combination of strawberry and chocolate, especially with crunchy streusel on top, but any flavor pairing will work.

MAKES ONE 9-INCH PIE

FOR THE CRUST

¼ cup coconut oil, solid, plus more for greasing the pan

2½ cups almond flour

3 tablespoons 100% unsweetened cacao powder

¾ cup plus 1 tablespoon arrowroot powder

Pinch of Himalayan pink salt

¼ cup maple syrup

1 large egg

FOR THE FILLING

1 quart Strawberry Ice Cream (page 229)

1 cup strawberries, sliced ⅛ inch thick

1 cup streusel (see page 77)

5 ounces 100% cacao unsweetened baking chocolate, melted

1. Preheat the oven to 350°F. Grease a 9-inch pie pan with coconut oil.

2. **MAKE THE CRUST:** In a medium bowl, whisk together the flour, cacao powder, arrowroot powder, and salt. Cut the coconut oil into the dry ingredients with a pastry blender or your fingertips until a dough comes together. It will look like wet sand, and the fats should be pea-size. Stir in the maple syrup and egg until fully incorporated. Gently shape the dough into a ball, cover with plastic wrap, press into a disk, and chill in the freezer for about 2 hours.

3. Roll out the dough about ¼ inch thick and 11-inches wide. Place in the pie pan by rolling the dough up around the rolling pin and gently placing in the pan. Trim any excess, and bake for about 10 minutes, until matte and firm to the touch. Allow it to cool completely.

4. **MAKE THE FILLING:** To make the ice cream extra easy to spread, whip it with an electric mixer for a minute or two until creamy and soft, but not melting. Immediately spread the ice cream into the cooled piecrust. Cover with plastic wrap and freeze for at least an hour, until set.

5. To serve, top the pie with fresh strawberries, streusel, and a drizzle of melted cacao. Eat immediately, or hold in the freezer for up to an hour with the toppings.

Note

Ice cream pie is even easier than ice cream cake. Any combination of piecrust and ice cream will work, and the crust and ice cream base will keep in your freezer indefinitely, ready to decorate at a moment's notice. Our graham cracker crust (see page 129) and coconut crust (see page 136) are both delicious options.

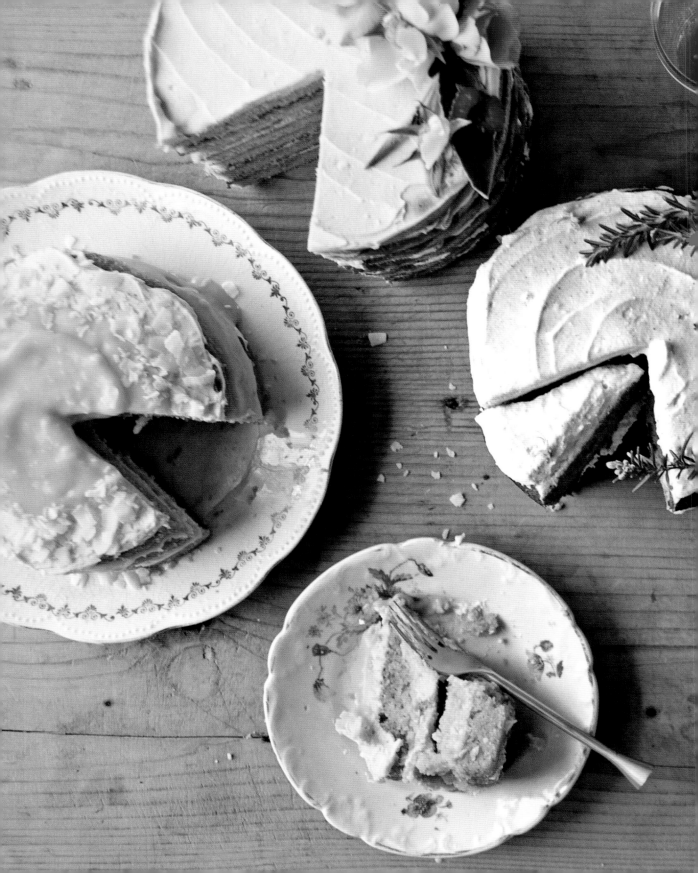

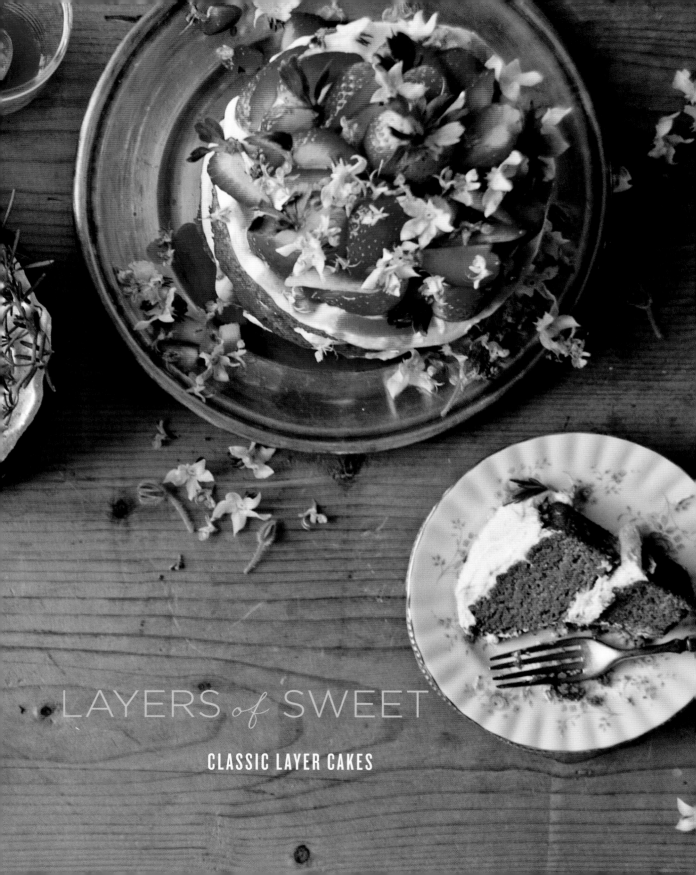

LAYERS of SWEET

CLASSIC LAYER CAKES

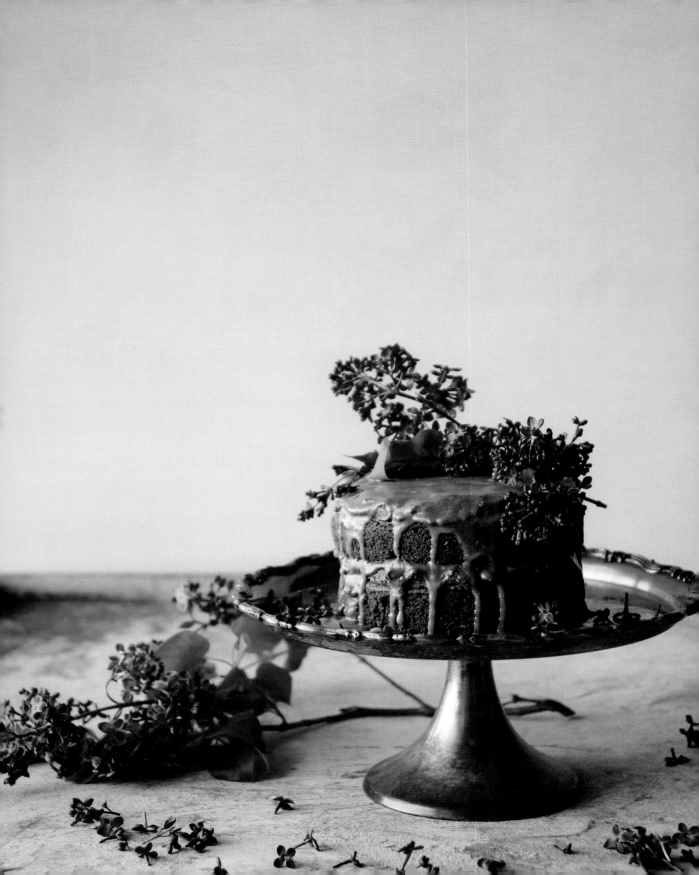

THE CHOCOLATE CAKE THAT CHANGED EVERYTHING

This was the cake that changed everything. Our whole company, and point of view, is founded on this cake. Decadent, rich, beautiful, and intensely chocolaty, it flies in the face of people who don't think you can have your cake and be grain-free, too. This cake is a showstopper, so get ready—people will freak out over it.

MAKES TWO 6-INCH LAYERS OR ONE 8-INCH CAKE

Coconut oil, for greasing the pans

2½ cups almond flour

¼ cup 100% unsweetened cacao powder

1 teaspoon baking soda

½ teaspoon Himalayan pink salt

2 large eggs

¾ cup maple syrup

1 tablespoon vanilla extract

1 cup Dark Chocolate Fudge Frosting (page 213)

1 cup Vegan Caramel (page 40), optional

1. Preheat the oven to 350°F. Line two 6-inch cake pans or one 8-inch cake pan with parchment paper rounds, then grease the sides of the pans with coconut oil.

2. In a medium bowl, whisk together the flour, cacao powder, baking soda, and salt. In a large bowl, whisk the eggs, maple syrup, and vanilla. A little at a time, add the dry ingredients to the wet, stirring until a batter forms.

3. Divide the batter evenly between the prepared pans and bake for about 25 minutes, or until a toothpick inserted into the center comes out clean. Invert the cakes onto racks and allow to cool completely.

4. Place one layer on a cake plate and top with ½ cup of the fudge frosting, smoothing it evenly over the entire surface. Drizzle ½ cup of the caramel on top, if using. Add the second cake layer and top with the remaining ½ cup frosting, then drizzle the remaining caramel over the cake, letting it drip down the sides. Refrigerate for 1 hour before serving.

VANILLA COCONUT JAM CAKE

This cake is a bestseller at Sweet Laurel Bakery, and it is no wonder why. Laurel created this recipe for her friend Clara, while planning her tea party–themed bridal shower. Laurel set out to create a cake recipe that was perfect alongside a cup of tea, and could also act as a centerpiece on each table. Each round of vanilla cake is sliced into two thin and delicate layers, stuffed with fresh berry jam and coconut whipped cream. After all, a tea party would not be complete without jam and cream!

MAKES THREE 6-INCH LAYERS OR TWO 8-INCH LAYERS

1 cup coconut oil, melted, plus more for greasing the pans

1 cup coconut flour

½ teaspoon baking soda

½ teaspoon Himalayan pink salt

1 cup maple syrup

8 large eggs

1 tablespoon vanilla extract

1 cup Coconut Whipped Cream (page 30)

1½ cups Berry Jam Filling (page 208) using raspberries

1. Preheat the oven to 350°F. Line three 6-inch cake pans or two 8-inch cake pans with parchment paper rounds, then grease the sides of the pans with coconut oil.

2. In a large bowl, whisk together the flour, baking soda, and salt. In a separate large bowl, combine the coconut oil, maple syrup, eggs, and vanilla. A little at a time, add the dry ingredients to the wet, stirring until a batter forms.

3. Divide the batter evenly among the prepared pans and bake for about 25 minutes, until a toothpick inserted into the center comes out clean. Invert the cakes onto racks and allow to cool completely.

4. Slice each cake round in half horizontally with a long serrated knife. Place one layer on a cake plate and top with 1 tablespoon of the raspberry jam, then 2 tablespoons of the coconut whipped cream, smoothing each evenly over the entire surface. Add another cake layer, and repeat. Continue until all layers have been used, and top the final layer with the remaining jam and coconut whipped cream. Refrigerate until ready to serve.

Note

Although you can make this cake without halving the layers, the cake is absolutely at its finest when you do.

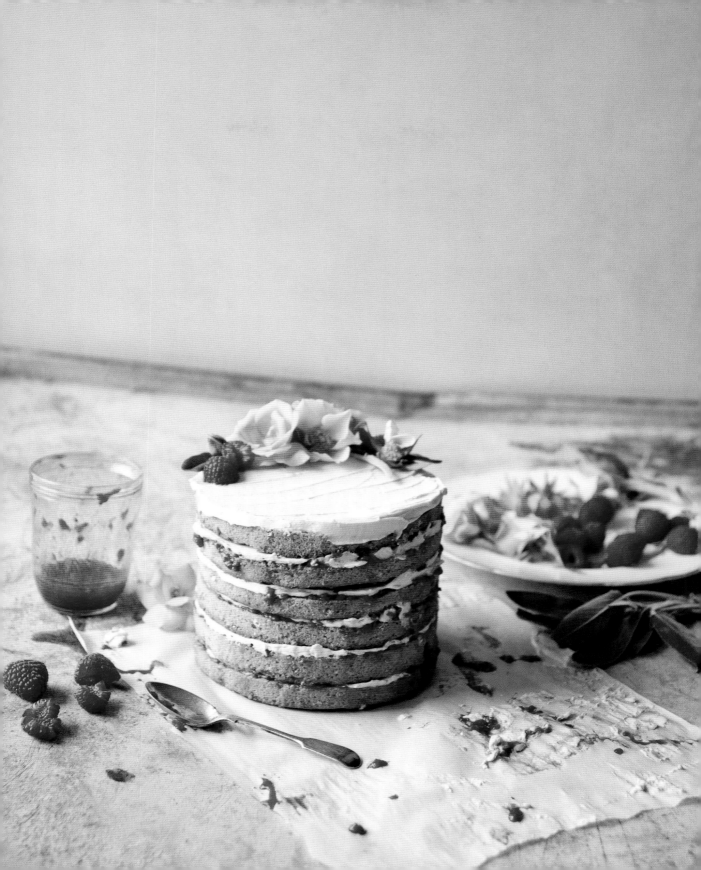

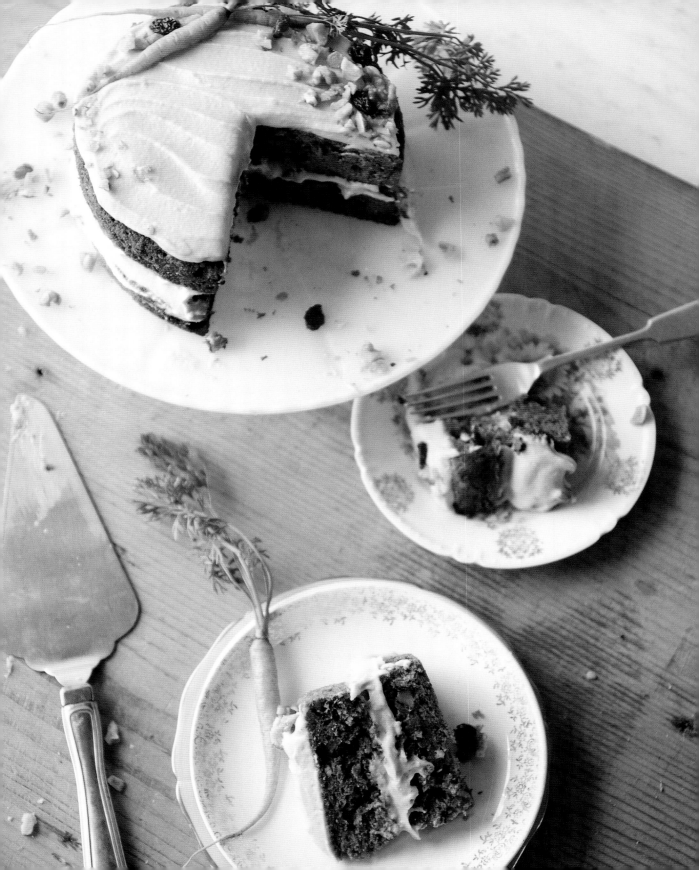

DARK HORSE CARROT CAKE
with PROBIOTIC CREAM CHEESE FROSTING

Claire is firmly on Team Chocolate Cake, but if Laurel had to choose her favorite Sweet Laurel cake, carrot cake is it! She loves this cake because it is lightly sweetened, allowing the carrots and raisins to be front and center. Although Laurel's husband, Nick, is the one usually eating cake for breakfast, even she will occasionally indulge in this one with her morning coffee. We call it the "dark horse" cake because it seems to be the unexpected favorite at so many of our cake tastings. Maybe it's the cinnamon scent, or the bright and creamy probiotic frosting we pair with it, or the whole package, but it's without a doubt a winner.

MAKES TWO 6-INCH LAYERS OR ONE 8-INCH CAKE

¼ cup coconut oil, melted, plus more for greasing the pans

2 cups almond flour

1 teaspoon baking soda

½ teaspoon Himalayan pink salt

1 tablespoon ground cinnamon

3 large eggs

⅓ cup maple syrup

1½ cups grated carrots

½ cup raisins

½ cup finely chopped walnuts

1 cup Probiotic Cream Cheese Frosting (page 208)

1. Preheat the oven to 350°F. Line two 6-inch cake pans or one 8-inch cake pan with parchment paper rounds, then grease the sides of the pans with coconut oil.

2. In a medium bowl, whisk together the flour, baking soda, salt, and cinnamon. In a large bowl, combine the eggs, maple syrup, and coconut oil. A little at a time, add the dry ingredients to the wet, stirring until a batter forms. Gently stir in the carrots, raisins, and walnuts.

3. Divide the batter evenly between the prepared pans and bake for about 30 minutes, or until a toothpick inserted into the center comes out clean. Invert the cakes onto racks and allow to cool completely.

4. Place one layer on a cake plate and top with ½ cup of the cream cheese frosting, smoothing it evenly over the entire surface. Add the second cake layer, top with another ½ cup frosting, and smooth the surface. For an 8-inch cake, you can cover the entire cake with the frosting. Refrigerate until ready to serve.

PUMPKIN SPICE LATTE CAKE

Even though Claire put her foot down and said, "No pumpkin bread. Every gluten-free bakery has one!" Laurel persisted. She snuck some onto the spread at a Sweet Laurel workshop and Claire literally ate her words, with vegan caramel on top. Now, every fall, people go nuts for our pumpkin bread. We knew we had to turn it into a cake. Just as moist as our bread, but spread with chai coconut whipped cream, this cake is especially perfect for the holidays. And if you want to turn this pumpkin spice latte combo into a pumpkin chai latte–inspired one, simply switch out the espresso for chai.

MAKES TWO 6-INCH LAYERS OR ONE 8-INCH CAKE

3 tablespoons coconut oil, melted, plus more for greasing the pans

1 cup pumpkin puree

½ cup maple syrup

2 large eggs

1 tablespoon vanilla extract

2 cups almond flour

1 tablespoon ground cinnamon

1 teaspoon ground ginger

1 teaspoon baking soda

½ teaspoon Himalayan pink salt

2 cups Espresso Coconut Whipped Cream (page 31)

1. Preheat the oven to 350°F. Line two 6-inch cake pans or one 8-inch cake pan with parchment paper rounds, then grease the sides of the pans with coconut oil.

2. In a large bowl, whisk together the coconut oil, pumpkin, maple syrup, eggs, and vanilla. In a medium bowl, whisk the flour, cinnamon, ginger, baking soda, and salt. A little at a time, add the dry ingredients to the wet, stirring until a batter forms.

3. Divide the batter evenly between the prepared pans and bake for about 30 minutes, until a toothpick inserted into the center comes out clean. Invert the cakes onto racks and allow to cool completely.

4. Place one layer on a cake plate and top with ½ cup of the coconut whipped cream, smoothing it evenly over the entire surface. For a 6-inch cake, add the second cake layer, top with another ½ cup whipped cream, and smooth the surface. One tablespoon at a time, add whipped cream to the sides, smoothing with an offset spatula. For an 8-inch cake, you can cover the entire cake with the coconut whipped cream. Refrigerate until ready to serve.

Note

This cake is also delightful topped with Chai Coconut Whipped Cream (page 31) and Vegan Caramel (page 40). A Sweet Laurel favorite!

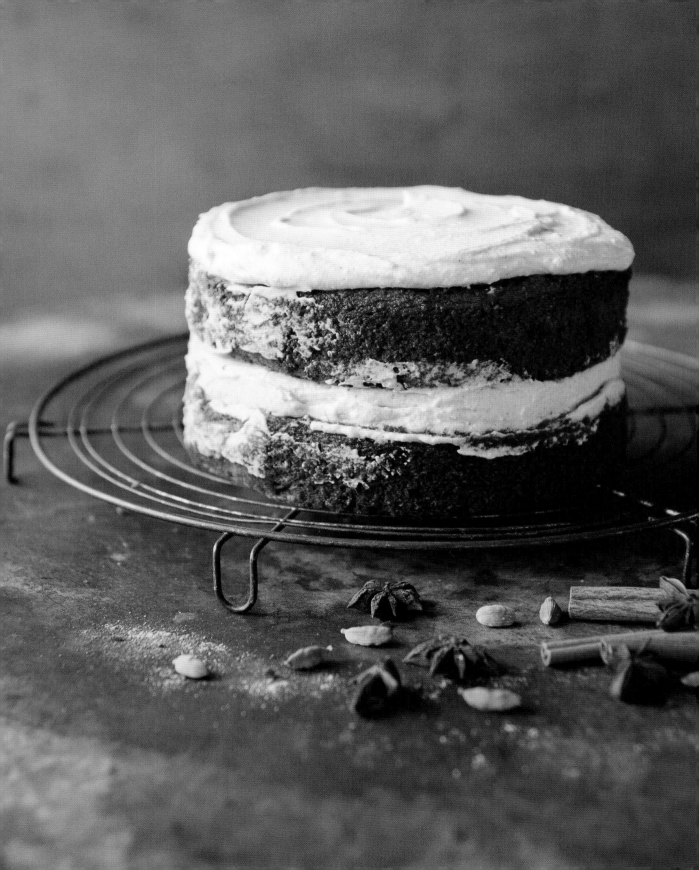

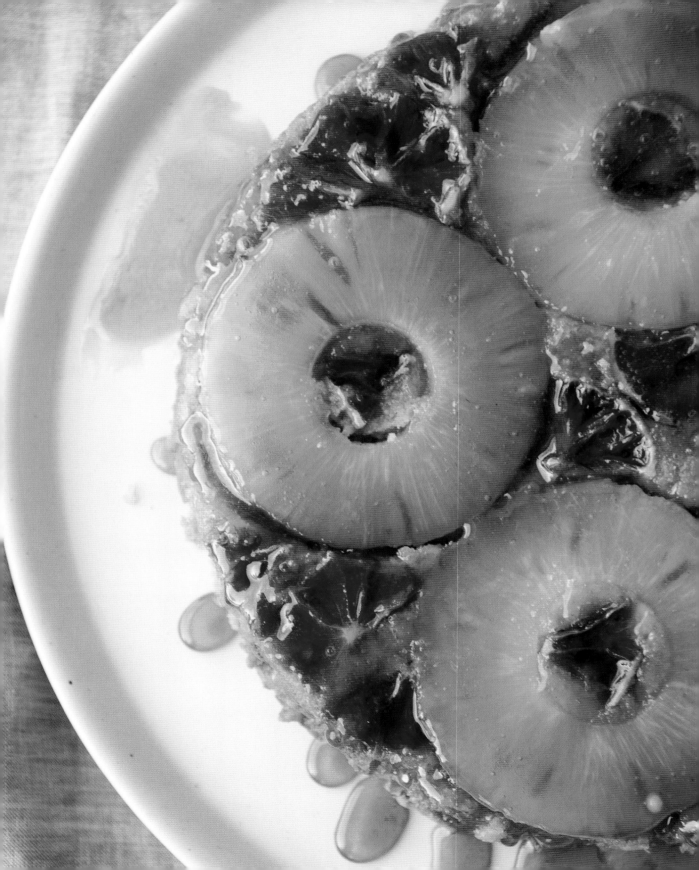

PINEAPPLE UPSIDE-DOWN CAKE

Who doesn't love a syrupy, warm, gorgeous cake? Claire grew up devouring her aunt Tina's classic pineapple upside-down cake for years, and it's one of her family's favorite recipes. Pineapple upside-down cake looks like a stained-glass window, with maraschino cherries dotting the glistening surface, and immediately sends us time traveling to the 1960s. For a more healthful option, we replaced maraschino cherries with slices of blood orange to get the same pop of brightness, and swapped the typical apricot jelly glaze for maple syrup to retain sweetness. With a cup of coffee in the afternoon, this is one of our favorite vintage-inspired treats.

MAKES ONE 9-INCH CAKE

¼ cup coconut oil, melted, plus more for greasing the pan

1 cup maple syrup

1 fresh pineapple, peeled, cored, and sliced into rounds ¼ inch thick, or 1 can sliced pineapple

1 blood orange, peeled and sliced into rounds

2 large eggs

1 tablespoon vanilla extract

2½ cups almond flour

½ teaspoon Himalayan pink salt

½ teaspoon baking soda

1. Preheat the oven to 350°F. Generously grease a 9-inch cake pan with coconut oil.

2. In a small saucepan over medium heat, bring ½ cup of the maple syrup to a simmer. Let it reduce for about 10 minutes, until thickened a bit, then set aside to cool slightly.

3. Arrange the pineapple in a circular pattern over the bottom of the prepared pan. Cover the gaps between the pineapple with the blood orange slices.

4. In a large bowl, whisk together the eggs, coconut oil, remaining ½ cup maple syrup, and vanilla. In a medium bowl, whisk the flour, salt, and baking soda. A little at a time, add the dry ingredients to the wet, stirring until a batter forms.

5. Pour the batter into the pan, completely covering the fruit, and bake for about 25 minutes, or until the center of the cake is firm to the touch. Quickly invert the cake onto a plate. Glaze with the reduced maple syrup and serve.

RICH FLOURLESS CHOCOLATE CAKE

By now, you've probably realized we have a bit of a chocolate habit at Sweet Laurel. Our flourless chocolate cake is so decadent, all you need is a sliver to satisfy even the most intense chocolate craving. It's like a truffle on a cake plate—dense, rich, and creamy. We like it best with piles of soft coconut whipped cream, perfect for cutting through the richness.

MAKES ONE 9-INCH CAKE

1 cup coconut oil, melted, plus more for greasing the pan

8 ounces 100% cacao unsweetened baking chocolate

½ cup date paste, store-bought or homemade (page 42)

½ cup 100% unsweetened cacao powder

1 cup maple syrup

2 tablespoons vanilla extract

8 large eggs

Coconut Whipped Cream (page 30), for serving

1. Preheat the oven to 350°F. Thoroughly grease a 9-inch springform pan with coconut oil.

2. In a medium saucepan over very low heat, melt the coconut oil and cacao together, stirring. The chocolate will melt very quickly, so be sure not to burn it. Once the mixture has melted, remove the pan from the heat and allow to cool completely.

3. Transfer the cooled cacao mixture to a blender. Add the date paste and blend until completely combined. Transfer the mixture to a medium bowl and whisk in the cacao powder, maple syrup, vanilla, and eggs until a batter forms. Pour the batter into the prepared pan and bake for 25 to 30 minutes, or until the edges are fully set (see Note). Let the cake cool in the pan for 10 minutes before sliding a knife around the edge and removing the sides. Let cool to room temperature. Serve with the coconut whipped cream. The cake will last on your counter for up to 2 days, or in the fridge for a week.

Note

The toothpick test does not work with this cake. You'll know it's done when the edges are fully set.

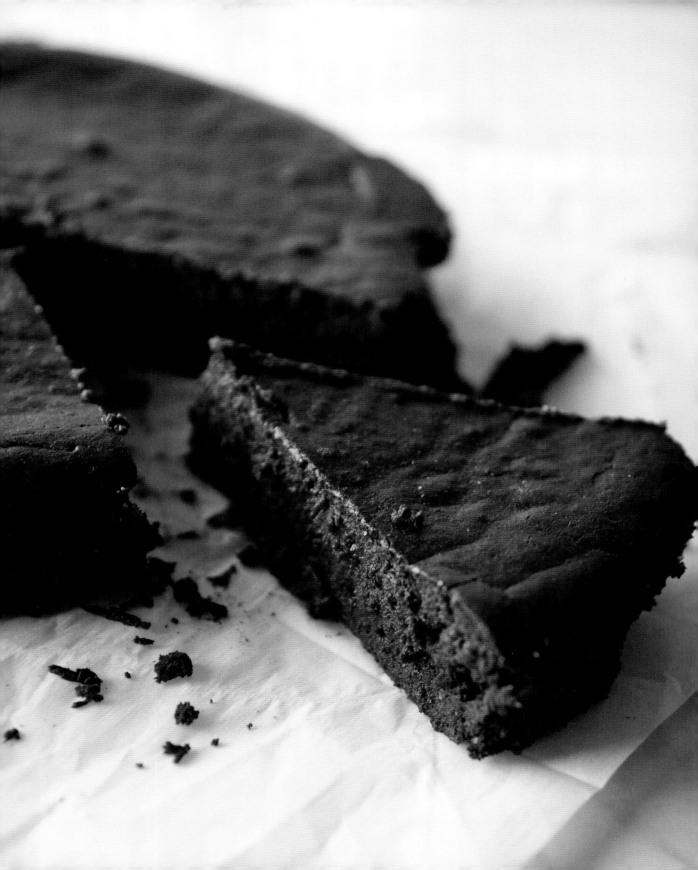

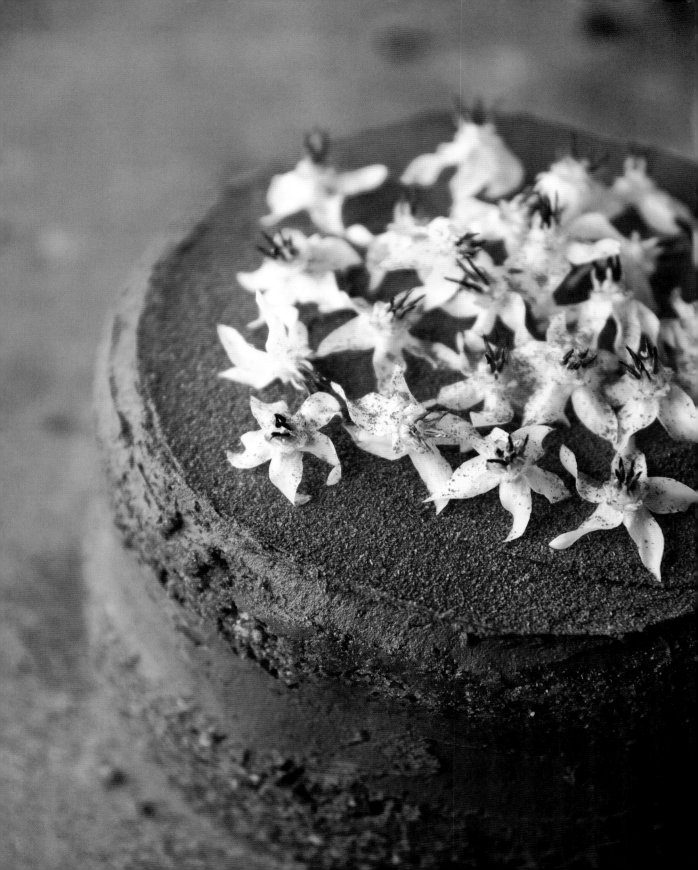

PECAN LAYER CAKE
with SPICY MEXICAN HOT CHOCOLATE GANACHE

One of our favorite bean-to-bar chocolate shops is down the street from our kitchen, and this cake is inspired by the owners' flavors of traditional Mexican chocolate. They take the cacao beans from their southern Mexican plantation and create the deepest, most nuanced chocolate we've ever had. Laurel keeps a bar in her purse at all times. Inspired by Mexican hot chocolate, this cake is spiced with cayenne and cinnamon and made with pecan flour. The lovely heat cuts through the mellow sweetness of the nuts. You can add as much or as little spice as you like, but we prefer this cake with a kick.

MAKES TWO 6-INCH LAYERS OR ONE 8-INCH CAKE

⅓ cup coconut oil, melted, plus more for greasing the pans

2 cups pecans

1 teaspoon baking soda

½ teaspoon ground cinnamon

½ teaspoon Himalayan pink salt

2 large eggs

½ cup maple syrup

1 tablespoon vanilla extract

1 cup Mexican Hot Chocolate Ganache (page 214)

1. Preheat the oven to 350°F. Line two 6-inch cake pans or one 8-inch cake pan with parchment paper rounds, then grease the sides of the pans with coconut oil.

2. In a food processor, pulse the pecans until they reach the consistency of nut flour. Be careful not to pulse too much, or it will turn into nut butter. Transfer to a medium bowl and whisk together with the baking soda, cinnamon, and salt. In a large bowl, combine the coconut oil, eggs, maple syrup, and vanilla. A little at a time, add the dry ingredients to the wet, stirring until a batter forms.

3. Divide the batter evenly between the prepared pans and bake for about 30 minutes, until a toothpick inserted into the center comes out clean. Invert the cakes onto racks and allow to cool completely.

4. Place one layer on a cake plate and top with ½ cup of the ganache, smoothing it evenly over the entire surface. Add the second cake layer, top with another ½ cup ganache, and smooth. For an 8-inch cake, you can cover the entire cake with the ganache. Refrigerate until ready to serve.

PINK STRAWBERRY LAYER CAKE

What could be more darling than a blush-pink cake, piled high with strawberries and cream? Sometimes inspiration for us comes from a visual cue rather than a flavor or texture, and in this case, it was pink. We wanted to create something rosy and ultrafeminine, almost like the inside-out version of our Vanilla Coconut Jam Cake (page 168). We love late spring strawberries for this cake, but feel free to try a magenta version with raspberries, or purple with blackberries.

MAKES THREE 6-INCH LAYERS OR TWO 8-INCH LAYERS

¼ cup coconut oil, melted, plus more for greasing the pans

4 cups almond flour

1 teaspoon baking powder

½ teaspoon Himalayan pink salt

3 cups strawberries, hulled, plus 1 cup quartered strawberries

¼ cup roughly chopped raw beets

⅔ cup honey (maple syrup works as well, but we use honey so the pink color comes through)

5 large eggs

3 tablespoons fresh lemon juice

2 tablespoons apple cider vinegar

1 tablespoon vanilla extract

1 cup Berry Jam Filling (page 208) using strawberries

2 cups Coconut Whipped Cream (page 30)

1. Preheat the oven to 350°F. Line three 6-inch cake pans or two 8-inch cake pans with parchment paper rounds, then grease the sides of the pans with coconut oil.

2. In a large bowl, whisk together the flour, baking powder, and salt. Pulse the hulled strawberries in a blender or food processor until mashed. Add the beets, honey, coconut oil, eggs, lemon juice, vinegar, and vanilla, and pulse again to combine. Add the flour mixture and blend until completely smooth.

3. Divide the batter evenly between the prepared pans and bake for 30 to 40 minutes, until a toothpick inserted into the center comes out clean. Invert the cakes onto racks and allow to cool completely.

4. While the cakes cool, cook down the strawberry jam in a medium saucepan over medium heat until it just reaches a syrup consistency.

5. Place one layer on a cake plate and top with ½ cup of the coconut whipped cream, smoothing it evenly over the entire surface. Then add ¼ cup of jam. Add the second cake layer and top with another ½ cup whipped cream, and ¼ cup jam. Add the third layer and top with the remaining whipped cream, then drizzle the remaining thickened jam over the top, letting it run down the sides. Decorate with the quartered strawberries. For two 8-inch layers, do the same build of coconut whipped cream and jam, with the remaining jam drizzled over the top. Refrigerate until ready to serve.

_____ *Note* _____

When using natural dyes, like fruit, to give your cake a vibrant hue, it's not as simple as putting in some beet juice and calling it a day. To make the color stick, rather than turn brown, you have to add quite a bit of acid to "fix" the color to the cake. So be sure to follow the directions closely—no shortcuts this time!

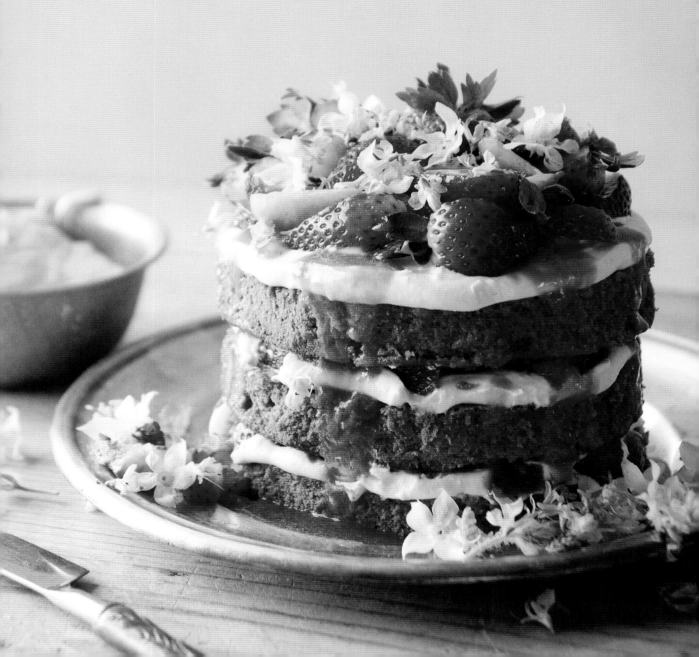

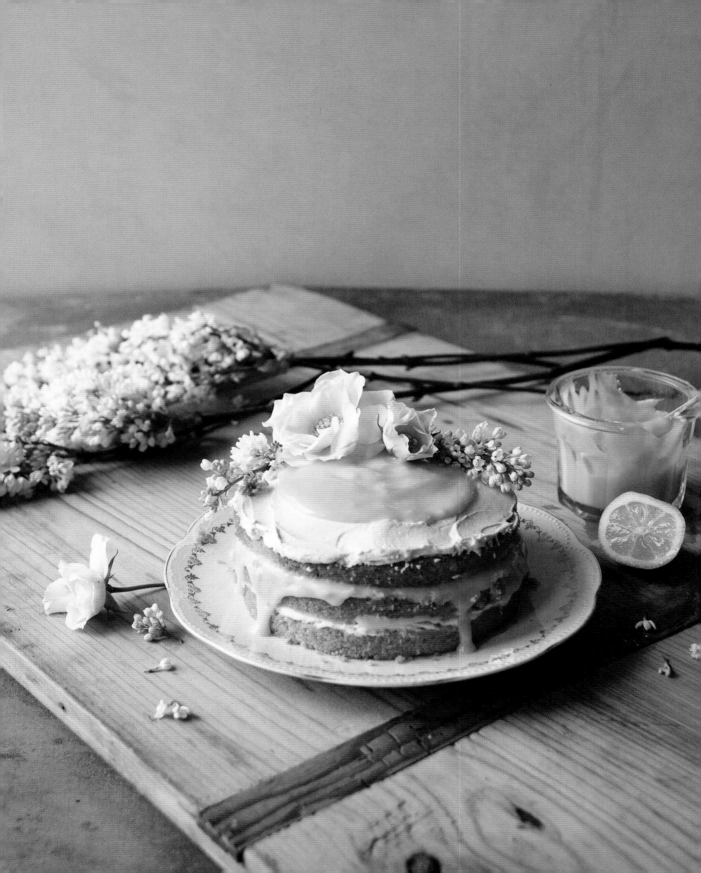

FLUFFY LEMON COCONUT CAKE

One of Laurel's strangest habits is her ability to eat lemons like apples. All through her pregnancy she found herself craving lemons. She created this recipe as an ode to her favorite citrus, so you can be sure the sharp brightness of lemon comes through in every bite. The lemon spread is our take on a lemon curd, and mixed with coconut whipped cream and a lemon-scented cake base, this dessert is heavenly. It was the perfect centerpiece to Laurel's citrus-inspired baby shower.

MAKES THREE 6-INCH LAYERS OR TWO 8-INCH LAYERS

¼ cup coconut oil, melted, plus more for greasing the pans

2½ cups almond flour

1 teaspoon baking soda

½ teaspoon Himalayan pink salt

2 large eggs

½ cup maple syrup

¼ cup fresh lemon juice

Grated zest of 1 lemon

¼ cup unsweetened flaked coconut

2 cups Coconut Whipped Cream (page 30)

1 cup Lemon Spread (page 222)

1. Preheat the oven to 350°F. Line three 6-inch cake pans or two 8-inch cake pans with parchment paper rounds, then grease the sides of the pans with coconut oil.

2. In a medium bowl, whisk together the flour, baking soda, and salt. In a large bowl, whisk together the eggs, coconut oil, maple syrup, lemon juice, and zest. A little at a time, add the dry ingredients to the wet, stirring until a batter forms.

3. Divide the batter evenly between the prepared pans and bake for about 30 minutes, until a toothpick inserted into the center comes out clean. Invert the cakes onto racks and allow to cool completely.

4. Spread the coconut flakes over the lined baking sheet and put in the still-hot oven for about 10 minutes, or until fragrant and just golden brown. Remove and set aside to cool.

5. Place one layer on a cake plate and top with 2 tablespoons of the lemon spread and ½ cup of the coconut whipped cream, smoothing each evenly over the entire surface. Add another cake layer, and repeat. Continue until all layers have been used, and top the cake with the remaining whipped cream and lemon spread. Finish with a sprinkling of toasted coconut. For two 8-inch layers, do the same build of coconut whipped cream and lemon spread, with the lemon spread and toasted coconut sprinkled on top. Refrigerate until ready to serve.

PISTACHIO ROSE CAKE
with PINK ROSE BUTTERCREAM

One of our dear friends has an almond allergy, which meant Laurel would have to improvise if she wanted to bring her a baked treat. Hazelnut or coconut flour is our typical backup plan if someone is allergic to almonds, but one day Laurel found pistachio flour at our favorite neighborhood health food store. She was instantly inspired. The combination of pistachio and rose is common in Middle Eastern cuisine; we love the blend of soft nuttiness with a whisper of floral.

MAKES TWO 6-INCH LAYERS OR ONE 8-INCH CAKE

¼ cup coconut oil, melted, plus more for greasing the pans

2 cups pistachio flour or finely ground raw pistachios (see Note)

½ cup almond or hazelnut flour

½ teaspoon Himalayan pink salt

1 teaspoon baking soda

2 large eggs

½ cup maple syrup

1 teaspoon vanilla extract

2 cups Pink Rose Buttercream (page 209)

Shelled pistachios, for garnish

1. Preheat the oven to 350°F. Line two 6-inch cake pans or one 8-inch cake pan with parchment paper rounds, then grease the sides of the pans with coconut oil.

2. In a large bowl, whisk together the pistachio flour, almond flour, salt, and baking soda. In a medium bowl, whisk the eggs, coconut oil, maple syrup, and vanilla. A little at a time, add the dry ingredients to the wet, stirring until a batter forms.

3. Divide the batter evenly between the cake pans and bake for 25 to 30 minutes, until a toothpick inserted into the center comes out clean. Invert the cakes onto racks, and allow to cool completely.

4. Slice each cake round in half horizontally. Place one layer on a cake plate and top with ¼ cup of the buttercream, smoothing it evenly over the entire surface. Add another cake layer and repeat. Continue until all layers have been used, and top with the remaining buttercream. For the 8-inch layer cake, cover entirely with buttercream. Refrigerate until ready to serve. Sprinkle with pistachios just before serving.

Note

If you can't find pistachio flour, you can make your own by grinding raw pistachios in a food processor. But be careful! If you overgrind them, you'll end up with pistachio butter rather than pistachio flour.

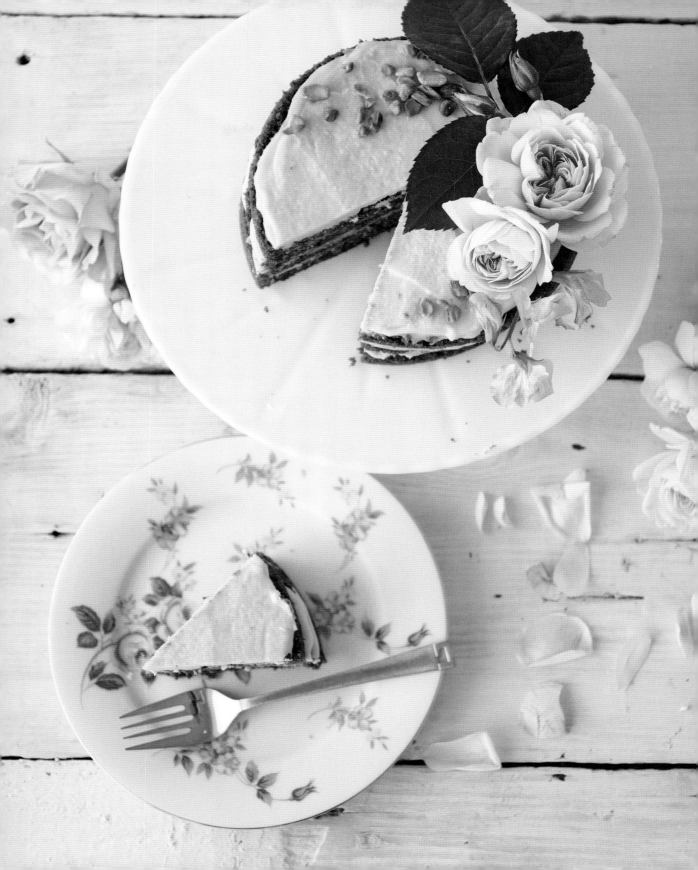

This recipe is best with a vegan caramel drizzle, rather than the thicker, spreadable caramel. Be sure to use the thinner option, as described in the Note on page 40.

TRES LECHES CAKE

It's impossible not to have a soft spot for a slice of this sweet cake sitting in a puddle of milk. The presentations vary. Some are incredibly sweet, some are dotted with maraschino cherries, and some, like ours, are stacked high. Our version swaps the classic sweetened condensed milk, evaporated milk, and cream for almond milk, hazelnut or pecan milk, and coconut milk. We filled the layers with simple coconut whipped cream, and devoured it almost immediately. Remember: Do not fear the puddle. The puddle of milk in the cake dish is a sign of a true tres leches cake. Because this cake needs to soak in the milks, it takes a little longer to assemble, so be sure to budget for the extra time.

MAKES TWO 6-INCH LAYERS OR ONE 8-INCH CAKE

Coconut oil, for greasing the pans

1 cup almond milk

1 cup hazelnut or pecan milk

1 cup full-fat coconut milk

FOR THE CAKE

1 cup coconut flour

½ teaspoon baking soda

½ teaspoon Himalayan pink salt

1 cup coconut oil, melted

1 cup maple syrup

8 large eggs

1 tablespoon vanilla extract

2 cups Coconut Whipped Cream (page 30)

½ cup Vegan Caramel (page 40)

1. Preheat the oven to 350°F. Line two 6-inch cake pans or one 8-inch cake pan with parchment paper rounds, then grease the sides of the pans with coconut oil.

2. Combine the three milks for soaking in a medium bowl and set aside.

3. **MAKE THE CAKE:** In a medium bowl, whisk together the coconut flour, baking soda, and salt. In another medium bowl, stir together the coconut oil, maple syrup, eggs, and vanilla. A little at a time, add the dry ingredients to the wet, stirring until a batter forms. Divide among the prepared pans.

4. Bake for 25 to 30 minutes, until a toothpick inserted into the center comes out clean. Invert the cakes onto racks and allow to cool completely. Poke the cakes with a fork all over to create holes for the tres leches to sink in.

5. Place the two layers in a 9 × 13-inch pan and pour the milk mixture over them. Let them sit overnight in the fridge.

6. Place one layer on a cake plate, drizzle with a few tablespoons of unabsorbed milk, and top with 1 cup of the coconut whipped cream, spreading it evenly. Add the second cake layer, drizzle with a few tablespoons of unabsorbed milk, and top with the remaining whipped cream, spreading evenly. Drizzle with the caramel. For the one 8-inch layer, drizzle with a few tablespoons of unabsorbed milk, spread entirely with the coconut whipped cream, and drizzle with caramel. Refrigerate until ready to serve.

BEET RED VELVET CAKE
with PROBIOTIC CREAM CHEESE FROSTING

This cake is our take on the classic red velvet cake with cream cheese frosting. Shunning the bottle of red food coloring, we looked to beets to color this rich red velvet cake. But here's the thing about baking with beets: the batter can look amazing, and then the cake turns a sad drab brown, while tasting very . . . beet-y. The trick is to lock in the color and balance the flavors to create a scarlet cake with a rich but not overly earthy flavor. The fresh beet must be paired with an acid; we chose apple cider vinegar and lemon juice.

MAKES THREE 6-INCH LAYERS OR TWO 8-INCH LAYERS

Coconut oil, for greasing the pans

4 cups almond flour

1 teaspoon baking soda

½ teaspoon Himalayan pink salt

2 tablespoons 100% unsweetened cacao powder

1 cup diced raw beets

¾ cup honey

3 large eggs

1 tablespoon apple cider vinegar

2 tablespoons fresh lemon juice

1 tablespoon vanilla extract

2 cups Probiotic Cream Cheese Frosting (page 208)

1. Preheat the oven to 350°F. Line three 6-inch cake pans or two 8-inch cake pans with parchment paper rounds, then grease the sides of the pans with coconut oil.

2. In a large bowl, whisk together the flour, baking soda, salt, and cacao powder. In a food processor or blender, puree the beets with the honey until smooth. Add the eggs and continue to blend. Add the vinegar, lemon juice, and vanilla and blend until combined. Pour into the dry ingredients and stir until a batter forms.

3. Divide the batter evenly between the prepared pans and bake for 30 to 40 minutes, or until a toothpick inserted into the center comes out clean. Invert the cakes onto racks and allow to cool completely.

4. Place one layer on a cake plate and top with ½ cup of the frosting. Smooth over the entire surface. Add the second cake layer and top with another ½ cup frosting. Repeat with the third cake layer. Smooth evenly over the surface. One tablespoon at a time, add frosting to the sides, smoothing with an offset spatula. Refrigerate until ready to serve.

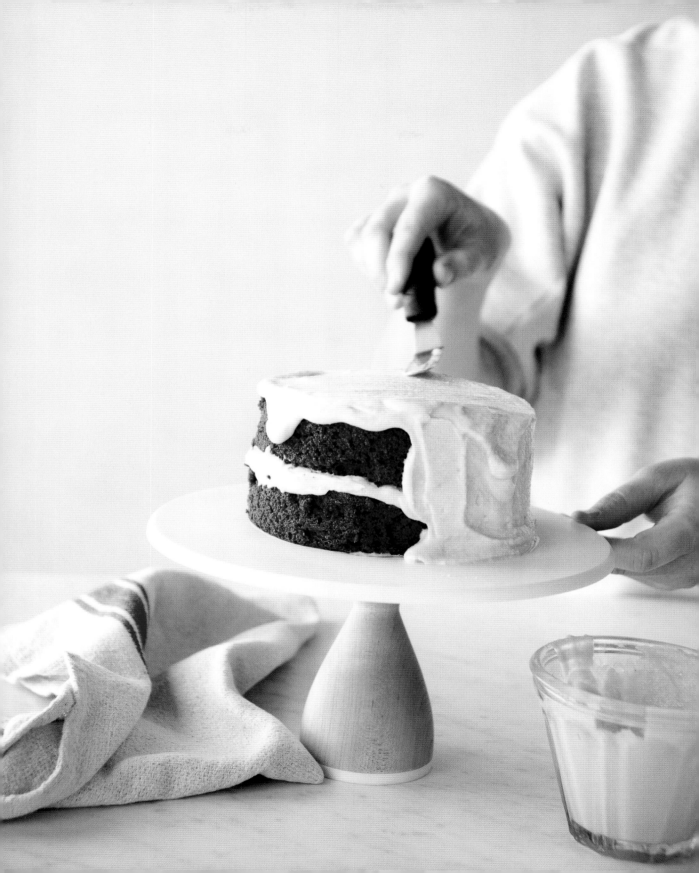

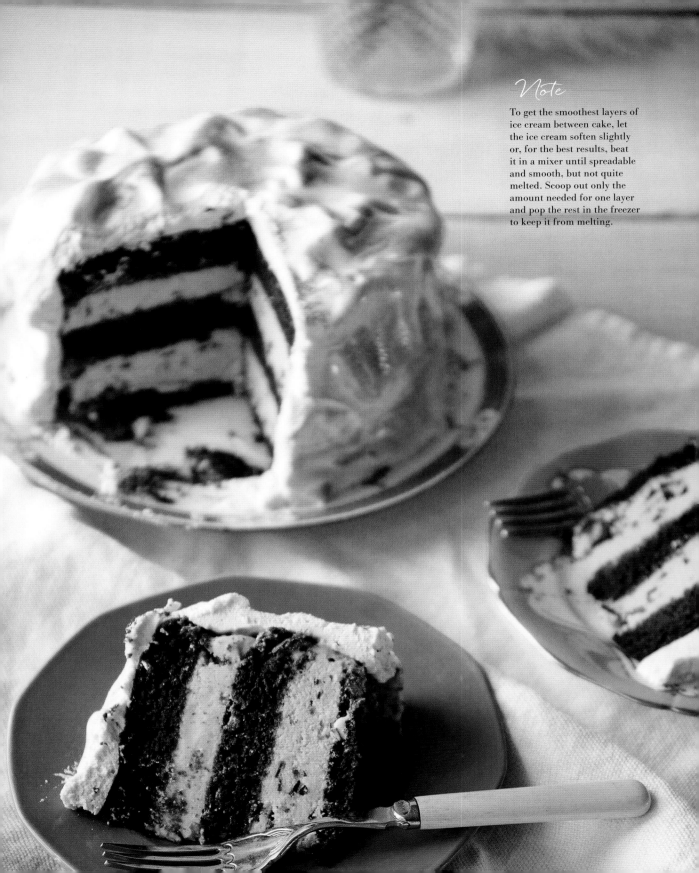

Note

To get the smoothest layers of ice cream between cake, let the ice cream soften slightly or, for the best results, beat it in a mixer until spreadable and smooth, but not quite melted. Scoop out only the amount needed for one layer and pop the rest in the freezer to keep it from melting.

MINT CHOCOLATE CHIP ICE CREAM CAKE
with MARSHMALLOW FROSTING

Laurel had mint chocolate chip ice cream cake for nearly every birthday party growing up. We both love this flavor of ice cream, and paired with layers of chocolate cake and decadent marshmallow topping, this dessert is totally irresistible, even now that we're all grown up. If you're using marshmallow frosting, the cake must be served within 2 hours, as this frosting doesn't freeze well. If you're making this cake in advance, try ganache or buttercream, which keeps in the freezer.

MAKES THREE 6-INCH LAYERS OR TWO 8-INCH LAYERS

Coconut oil, for greasing the pans

2½ cups almond flour

¼ cup 100% unsweetened cacao powder

1 teaspoon baking soda

½ teaspoon Himalayan pink salt

2 large eggs

¾ cup maple syrup

1 tablespoon vanilla extract

Dairy-Free Mint Ice Cream (page 230), softened

Marshmallow Frosting (page 217)

1. Preheat the oven to 350°F. Line three 6-inch cake pans or two 8-inch cake pans with parchment paper rounds, then grease the pans with coconut oil.

2. In a large bowl, whisk together the flour, cacao powder, baking soda, and salt. In a medium bowl, whisk the eggs, maple syrup, and vanilla. Add the dry ingredients to the wet and stir until a batter forms.

3. Divide the batter evenly between the prepared pans and bake for 20 to 25 minutes, until firm to the touch and a toothpick inserted into the center comes out clean. Invert the cakes onto racks and allow to cool completely.

4. Line two cake pans the size of your cakes with plastic wrap, letting the excess hang over. Place one cake layer into a lined pan. Top with ¾ cup of the ice cream and spread evenly with an offset spatula. Add the second cake layer and repeat. Top with the last layer of cake and cover with the other lined pan (it should look like two clam-shelled cake pans). Chill in the freezer for about 2 hours to set.

5. No more than 2 hours before serving, coat the entire cake in marshmallow frosting (work quickly, as the frosting will set immediately on the frozen cake), using the back of a spoon to create decorative swoops. If not serving immediately, pop the cake in the freezer for no more than 2 hours. Then, if desired, toast the peaks of the marshmallow topping with a butane torch or (very carefully) singe them under the broiler.

APPLE GINGER CUPCAKES

Apples and sweet spices is one of our favorite combinations, and with the bright kick from ginger, these cupcakes are even more delicious. Alone, these cupcakes are perfect with a cup of tea, but topped with cinnamon-ginger coconut whipped cream, they're a simple but decadent dessert. The batter can also be baked into a loaf.

MAKES 12 CUPCAKES

3 tablespoons coconut oil, melted, plus more for greasing the pan

1 cup unsweetened applesauce, store-bought or homemade (page 29)

½ cup maple syrup

2 large eggs

1 tablespoon vanilla extract

2 cups almond flour

1 tablespoon ground ginger

1 teaspoon ground cinnamon

1 teaspoon baking soda

½ teaspoon Himalayan pink salt

2 cups Cinnamon-Ginger Coconut Whipped Cream (page 31)

1 apple, very thinly sliced, for garnish

Candied Ginger Syrup (page 221), for garnish

1. Preheat the oven to 350°F. Line 12 muffin cups with paper liners. Grease the top of the pan with coconut oil.

2. In a large bowl, whisk together the coconut oil, applesauce, maple syrup, eggs, and vanilla until smooth. In a medium bowl, whisk the flour, ginger, cinnamon, baking soda, and salt. A little at a time, add the dry ingredients to the wet, stirring until a batter forms.

3. Divide the batter evenly among the lined muffin cups and bake for 25 to 30 minutes, or until a toothpick inserted into the center comes out clean. Invert the cupcakes onto a rack, and allow to cool completely.

4. To serve, smooth a few tablespoons of the cinnamon-ginger whipped cream on top of each cupcake. Top with a few thin slices of apple and a drizzle of ginger syrup.

Note

You can also bake this as two 6-inch layers or one 8-inch layer if you want to turn it into a layer cake. Bake for 20 to 25 minutes, until golden brown. This trick works for all our cupcake recipes.

SWEDISH ALMOND CARAMEL CAKE

We draw on inspiration from so many places at Sweet Laurel: our childhoods, vintage cookbooks, the farmer's market, and in this case, photography. While clicking through Pinterest for recipe ideas, we came across this beauty—a Swedish almond caramel cake, studded heavily with crunchy almond slices. After learning more about this Nordic classic, we decided to give it the Sweet Laurel treatment, replacing the almond-scented butter cake base with a rich almond vanilla cake, and making our own crisp almond caramel topping by caramelizing maple syrup. It's dense, rich, and marvelously crunchy—the perfect cake to serve with a pot of tea.

MAKES ONE 9-INCH CAKE

FOR THE CAKE

½ cup coconut oil, melted, plus more for greasing the pan

3 large eggs

1 cup maple syrup

2 teaspoons vanilla extract

2 cups almond flour

2 tablespoons coconut flour

2 teaspoons baking powder

⅓ cup full-fat coconut milk

FOR THE TOPPING

½ cup coconut oil, solid

½ cup maple syrup

1 tablespoon arrowroot powder

2 tablespoons full-fat coconut milk

1 cup thinly sliced almonds

1. Preheat the oven to 350°F. Thoroughly grease a 9-inch springform pan with coconut oil.

2. **MAKE THE CAKE:** With an electric mixer, beat the eggs, maple, and vanilla until very light in color and texture, 2 to 3 minutes. In a medium bowl, whisk together the almond flour, coconut flour, and baking powder. A little at a time, stir the flour mixture into the egg mixture. Add the coconut oil and coconut milk and stir very gently until the batter is smooth. Pour the batter into the prepared pan and smooth the top with a spatula.

3. Bake for 30 to 35 minutes, until the cake is just set (to ensure it can hold up the topping). Meanwhile, prepare the topping.

4. **MAKE THE TOPPING:** Combine the coconut oil, maple syrup, arrowroot powder, coconut milk, and almonds in a medium saucepan over medium heat and simmer for 10 to 12 minutes, stirring continuously; the mixture should bubble and become slightly thicker. Remove from the heat right before pouring over the cake.

5. Spread the topping over the cake, still in the pan. Bake for an additional 15 to 20 minutes, until the topping is golden and bubbling.

6. Let the cake cool in the pan for 10 minutes before sliding a knife around the edge and removing the sides. Let cool to room temperature.

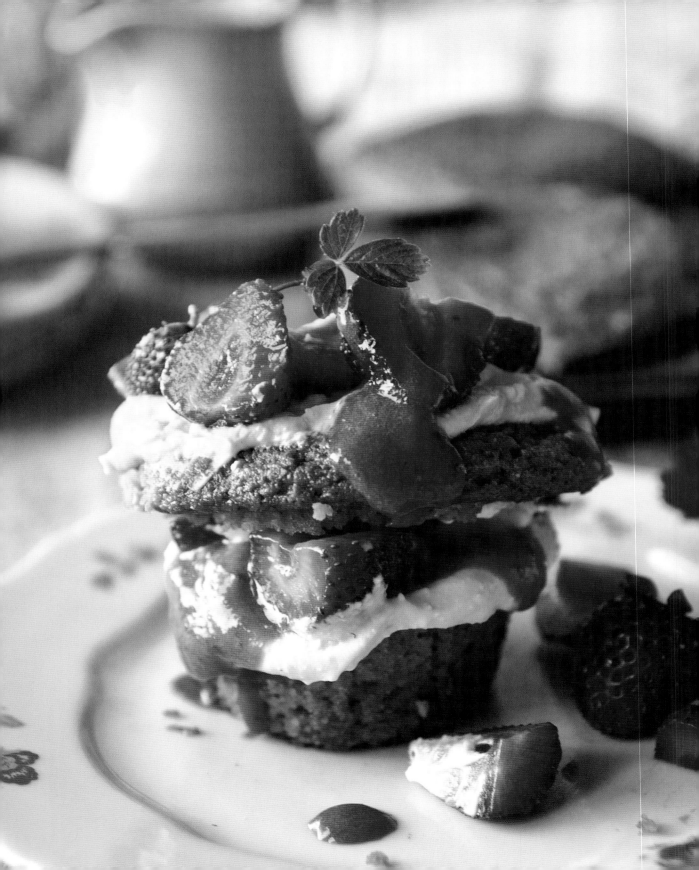

STRAWBERRY SHORTCAKE CUPCAKES

Growing up, we loved hosting afternoon tea for our dolls, and strawberry short-cakes would always make an appearance. They just seemed so perfectly dainty, and considering that the ingredients were always just cake, strawberries, and cream, they were easy to put together for our pretend table of guests. Even though the dolls were put away years ago, our love of strawberry shortcakes continues, especially served with our simple vanilla cupcakes and peak-of-season strawberries.

MAKES 9 CUPCAKES

2 cups almond flour

¼ teaspoon Himalayan pink salt

½ teaspoon baking soda

2 large eggs

½ cup full-fat coconut milk

½ cup maple syrup

1 pint strawberries, quartered

¼ cup raw honey

Juice of 1 lemon

Coconut Whipped Cream (page 30)

1. Preheat the oven to 350°F. Line 9 muffin cups with paper liners.

2. Whisk the flour, salt, and baking soda in a medium bowl. In a separate medium bowl, whisk together the eggs, coconut milk, and maple syrup until combined. A little at a time, add the dry ingredients to the wet, stirring until a batter forms.

3. Divide the batter evenly among the lined muffin cups and bake for 25 to 30 minutes, until golden brown and a toothpick inserted into the center comes out clean. Immediately invert onto a cooling rack. Allow the cupcakes to cool for about an hour.

4. To make the strawberry sauce, put 1 cup of the quartered strawberries, the honey, and lemon juice in a food processor and blend until completely smooth.

5. Cut off the top of each cupcake, add a spoonful of coconut whipped cream, some strawberries, and a touch of strawberry sauce. Add the cupcake top and repeat. Enjoy!

Note

We like to decorate our shortcakes by removing the tops of the cupcakes and creating two layers of cream and fruit, but you can keep it simple, just decorating the cupcake tops.

GERMAN CHOCOLATE CAKE

German chocolate is a classic American cake—like red velvet or hummingbird, people have a nostalgic reaction to it. For us, creating a grain-free version meant tapping into the flavors and textures we love about it—the rich chocolate flavor, the bit of brightness traditionally from buttermilk, the fluffy texture. This decadent cake is very similar to a devil's food cake, and is also brilliant with our toasted marshmallow frosting.

MAKES TWO 6-INCH LAYERS OR ONE 8-INCH CAKE

Coconut oil, for greasing the pans

2½ cups almond flour

1 teaspoon baking soda

½ teaspoon Himalayan pink salt

4 ounces 100% cacao unsweetened baking chocolate, melted

½ cup brewed coffee

3 large eggs

1 cup maple syrup

1 tablespoon apple cider vinegar

¼ cup coconut yogurt, store-bought or homemade (page 40)

1 tablespoon vanilla extract

2 cups Coconut Pecan Frosting (page 217)

Toasted coconut (see Note, page 137), for garnish

Pecan halves, for garnish

1. Preheat the oven to 350°F. Line two 6-inch cake pans or one 8-inch pan with parchment paper rounds, then grease the sides of the pans with coconut oil.

2. In a medium bowl, whisk together the flour, baking soda, and salt. In a large bowl, whisk the cacao, coffee, eggs, maple syrup, vinegar, coconut yogurt, and vanilla until well blended. A little at a time, add the dry ingredients to the wet, stirring to create a smooth batter.

3. Divide the batter evenly between the prepared pans and bake for 35 to 40 minutes, or until a toothpick inserted into the center comes out clean. Invert the cakes onto a rack and allow to cool completely while you prepare the frosting.

4. To build the cake, slice the cake layers in half horizontally, creating four layers. Place one layer on a cake plate and smooth ½ cup of the frosting over the entire surface. Add a second layer and spread with another ½ cup frosting. Continue with all four layers, spreading extra frosting on top. If making an 8-inch cake, slice in half, creating two layers, and serve with 1 cup of frosting spread on each layer. Garnish with toasted coconut and pecans.

OLIVE OIL CITRUS CUPCAKES
with DARK CHOCOLATE FUDGE FROSTING

Cupcakes usually make us think of classroom birthday parties, but with the sophisticated flavors of olive oil, citrus, and dark chocolate, it's impossible to think of these little cakes as anything but elegant.

MAKES 12 CUPCAKES

Coconut oil, for greasing the pan

4 cups almond flour

1½ teaspoons baking soda

½ teaspoon Himalayan pink salt

⅓ cup olive oil, plus more for drizzling

¾ cup maple syrup

2 tablespoons grated orange zest

¼ cup fresh orange juice

3 large eggs

Dark Chocolate Fudge Frosting (page 213)

Slices of dried orange peel, for garnish

1. Preheat the oven to 350°F. Line 12 muffin cups with paper liners. Grease the top of the pan with coconut oil.

2. In a medium bowl, whisk together the flour, baking soda, and salt. In a large bowl, whisk the olive oil, maple syrup, orange zest, orange juice, and eggs until smooth. A little at a time, add the dry ingredients to the wet, stirring until a batter forms.

3. Divide the batter evenly among the lined cups and bake for 25 to 30 minutes, until a toothpick inserted into the center comes out clean. Invert the cupcakes onto a rack and allow to cool completely.

4. Smooth 1 tablespoon of frosting on top of each cupcake. Top with a few thin slices of dried orange peel and a drizzle of olive oil.

Note

One of our favorite snacks is dried citrus slices. We make our own in a dehydrator, but they're also available at the farmer's market and in specialty stores.

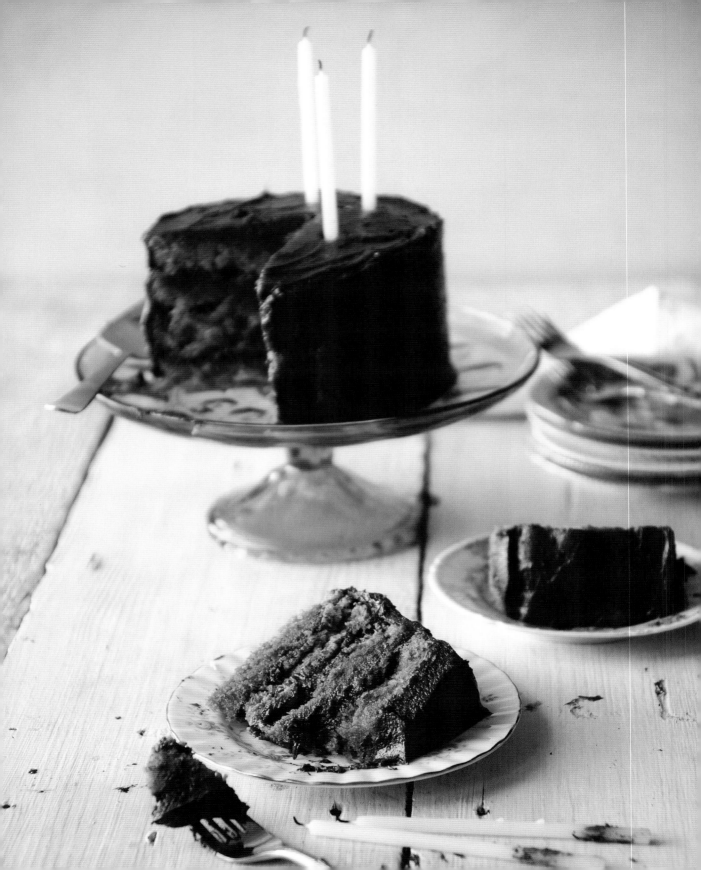

CLASSIC BIRTHDAY CAKE
with MILK CHOCOLATE FROSTING

Yellow birthday cake is one of our childhood favorites. Something about it immediately feels celebratory, especially when paired with creamy milk chocolate frosting. To get our cake perfectly golden, we add a touch of turmeric powder and get extra richness from an additional egg yolk.

MAKES TWO 6-INCH LAYERS OR ONE 8-INCH CAKE

½ cup coconut oil, melted, plus more for greasing the pans

2 large eggs plus 1 large egg yolk

¾ cup maple syrup

1 tablespoon vanilla extract

4 cups almond flour

1 teaspoon Himalayan pink salt

¼ teaspoon turmeric

1 teaspoon baking soda

2 cups Milk Chocolate Frosting (page 209)

1. Preheat the oven to 350°F. Line two 6-inch cake pans or one 8-inch cake pan with parchment paper rounds, then grease the sides of the pans with coconut oil.

2. In a large bowl, whisk together the eggs and yolk, coconut oil, maple syrup, and vanilla until well incorporated. In a medium bowl, whisk the flour, salt, turmeric, and baking soda until there are no clumps. Add the dry ingredients to the wet, stirring until a batter forms. Using a spatula, scoop the batter into the prepared pans and smooth out the tops.

3. Bake for 35 to 40 minutes, or until the cakes are golden brown and a toothpick inserted into the center comes out clean. Allow the cakes to cool completely before removing from the pan.

4. You can leave the cake in two layers or slice each layer in half horizontally, creating four (which we prefer, to maximize the cake-to-frosting ratio). To save for later, wrap each cake layer in plastic and refrigerate for up to 3 days; any longer and the turmeric might turn dark red as it oxidizes. For decorating four layers, place one layer on a cake plate and top with ¼ cup of the frosting, smoothing it evenly over the entire surface. Add the next cake layer, top with another ¼ cup frosting, and smooth. Repeat for all of the layers, then coat the cake with the remaining 1 cup frosting, smoothing it evenly all over. For an 8-inch cake, you can cover the entire cake with the frosting. Refrigerate until ready to serve.

—— *Note* ——

The small amount of turmeric in this recipe won't add any flavor—just color—but if you prefer, you can leave it out.

STICKY TOFFEE PUDDING

Few things smell as good as a kitchen halfway through the making of a sticky toffee pudding. The warm dates and vanilla, the maple syrup reducing, apples caramelizing in the oven—these golden smells will perfume your entire house and make it practically impossible to wait for the pudding to cool before devouring it. We added a stack of roasted apples on top, which give the pudding a delicious brightness in every bite.

SERVES 8

FOR THE PUDDING

¼ cup coconut oil, solid, plus more for greasing the dish

Arrowroot powder, for dusting the dish

8 ounces whole Medjool dates

½ cup boiling water

1 teaspoon vanilla extract

⅔ cup almond flour

1 teaspoon baking soda

¼ teaspoon Himalayan pink salt

⅔ cup maple syrup

2 large eggs

½ cup unsweetened applesauce, store-bought or homemade (page 29)

1. Preheat the oven to 350°F. Grease a 6-cup soufflé dish with coconut oil and coat with arrowroot powder, shaking to discard any excess.

2. **MAKE THE PUDDING:** Remove the pits and dice the dates. Put them in a medium bowl and cover with the boiling water. Let the dates soak for about 30 minutes, until room temperature, and then mash slightly with a fork. Stir in the vanilla.

3. While the dates are soaking, in a medium bowl, whisk together the flour, baking soda, and salt. With an electric mixer, beat the coconut oil and maple syrup together for a few minutes, until thick and smooth. Add the eggs one at a time, beating well after each one. Gently fold in one-third of the flour mixture, then half the applesauce. Repeat until all the flour and applesauce are used. Stir the soaked dates and their liquid (it should be mostly soaked into the dates) into the pudding batter. Spread it evenly into the dish and bake for 50 to 60 minutes, until risen and firm.

FOR THE SAUCE

1 cup maple syrup

¼ cup full-fat coconut milk

1 tablespoon vanilla extract

1 pinch Himalayan pink salt

FOR THE ROASTED APPLES

3 apples, peeled, cored, and cut into quarters

¼ cup maple syrup

1 tablespoon coconut oil, melted

4. **MAKE THE SAUCE:** Put the maple syrup in a medium saucepan over medium heat and bring to a boil, stirring constantly, for 10 minutes. Stir in the coconut milk, raise the heat slightly, and let the mixture reduce for 10 to 15 minutes, until you have a thick syrup. Remove from the heat and stir in the vanilla and salt. Set aside. If the sauce hardens, just heat it up again to make it liquid.

5. **MAKE THE ROASTED APPLES:** Preheat the oven to 425°F. Line a baking sheet with parchment paper. In a large bowl, combine the apples, maple syrup, and coconut oil, stirring to coat the fruit. Spread the apples over the baking sheet and bake for 25 to 30 minutes, until tender and caramelized.

6. Remove the pudding from the oven. It should be quite puffy, but it will collapse a bit as it cools. Leave it in the dish for a few minutes, and then loosen it with a small knife before turning it out onto a serving plate. Top with roasted apples and drizzle with sauce. This is best served warm, and is even better heated up the next day.

Note

This pudding is marvelous as a large cake, but it can easily be made in individual ramekins as well. Simply bake in eight deep 8-ounce ramekins for 20 to 30 minutes.

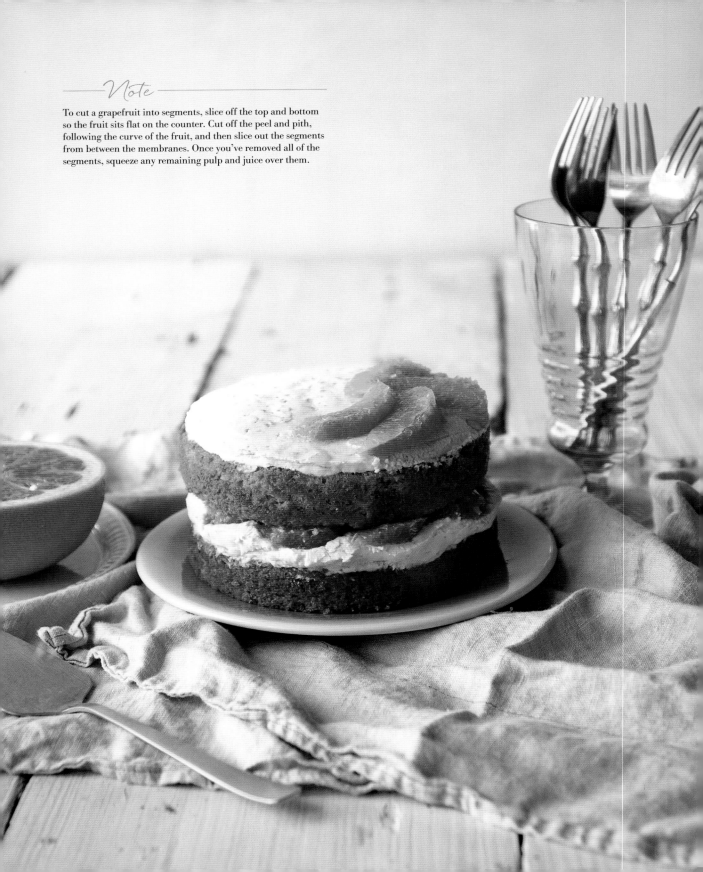

GRAPEFRUIT CAKE

Our shared love of Los Angeles history, along with our love of baking, formed the foundation of our friendship, so it should be no surprise that a historic LA cake made it into this chapter. The Brown Derby, a famous Hollywood watering hole to the stars, created a unique grapefruit cake with a simple sponge, crushed grapefruit, and grapefruit frosting. Inspired by the bright California citrus flavors, we created our own version, filled with fresh grapefruit and grapefruit-scented coconut cream. The key is to use the pinkest grapefruit you can find, but you can also try this recipe with other citrus, like blood oranges or sweet oro blanco grapefruit. The combination of sweet, tart, and just a touch bitter makes this cake a delicious throwback.

MAKES TWO 6-INCH LAYERS OR ONE 8-INCH LAYER

Coconut oil, for greasing the pans

2 cups almond flour

¼ teaspoon Himalayan pink salt

½ teaspoon baking soda

2 large eggs, separated

¼ cup full-fat coconut milk

½ cup maple syrup

1 tablespoon grated grapefruit zest

2 tablespoons grapefruit juice

1½ cups Grapefruit Coconut Whipped Cream (page 31)

2 grapefruits, cut into segments, for garnish

1. Preheat the oven to 350°F. Line two 6-inch cake pans or one 8-inch cake pan with parchment paper rounds, then grease the sides of the pans with coconut oil.

2. In a medium bowl, whisk the flour, salt, and baking soda. In a large bowl, whisk together the egg yolks, coconut milk, maple syrup, grapefruit zest, and grapefruit juice until combined. In another medium bowl, whisk the egg whites until soft peaks form, about 5 minutes with an electric mixer. Fold the egg whites into the egg yolk mixture. Gradually add the dry ingredients to the wet, folding to combine.

3. Divide the batter between the prepared pans and bake for 25 to 35 minutes, until the tops are golden brown and a toothpick inserted into the center comes out clean. Allow the cakes to cool in the pans for about an hour, then invert onto a rack to cool.

4. To build the cake, place one layer on a plate and top with ¾ cup of the coconut whipped cream. Smooth over the entire surface. Top with grapefruit segments. Add a second layer and top with another ¾ cup coconut whipped cream. Smooth over the surface and garnish with the remaining grapefruit segments.

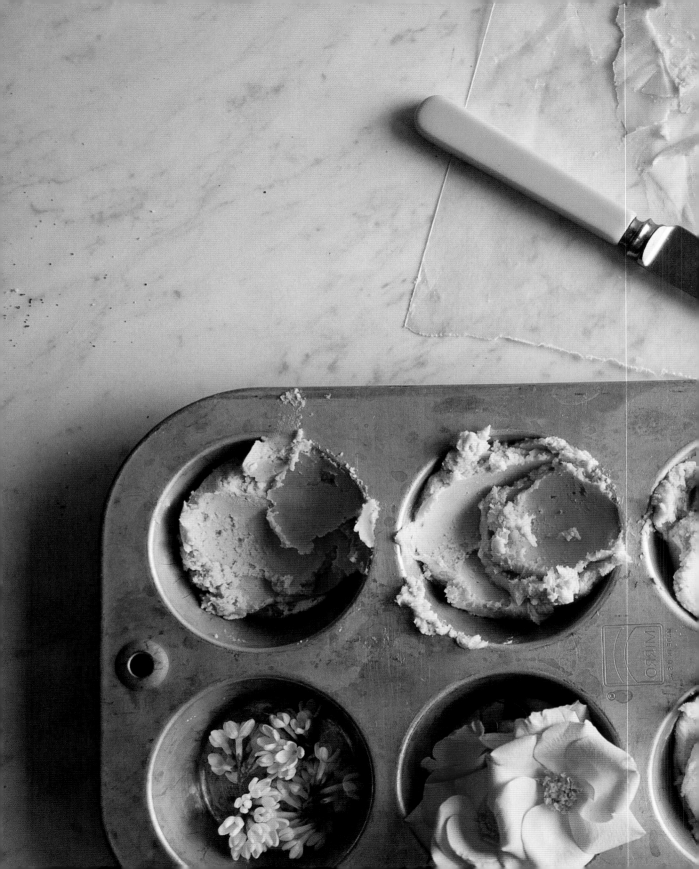

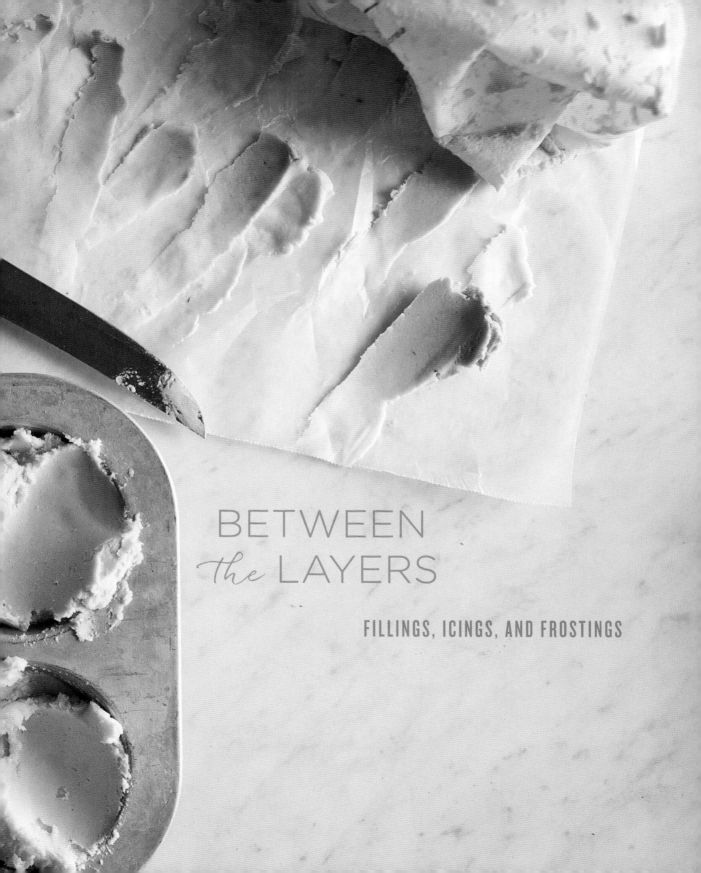

BETWEEN *the* LAYERS

FILLINGS, ICINGS, AND FROSTINGS

When Claire's grandmother was a little girl, at a fancy restaurant for her birthday dinner, she ordered a slice of chocolate cake. Knowing the dark chocolate frosting would be the best part, she ate all of the cake first, leaving the frosting to the end. Just as she lifted her fork to devour her plate of rich, buttery frosting, the server snatched it away, assuming she had eaten around the frosting because she didn't want it. There's a moral to this story: Stay vigilant when frosting is involved.

We love frosting at Sweet Laurel, and creamy, delicious, perfect frosting shouldn't rely on butter and sugar as its base. Instead, we turned to some of our favorite ingredients to make dairy-free and refined-sugar-free versions of your childhood favorites. We're featuring these special recipes in their own section to encourage you to mix, match, and experiment as you create your own cakes. For example, the Vanilla Coconut Jam Cake (page 168) can easily be filled with matcha-scented Coconut Buttercream (page 210) or our Lemon Spread (page 222) instead; The Chocolate Cake That Changed Everything (page 167) can be filled with airy Marshmallow Frosting (page 217) for a lighter option. This chapter offers many possibilities, and we hope you have fun discovering your own favorite combinations.

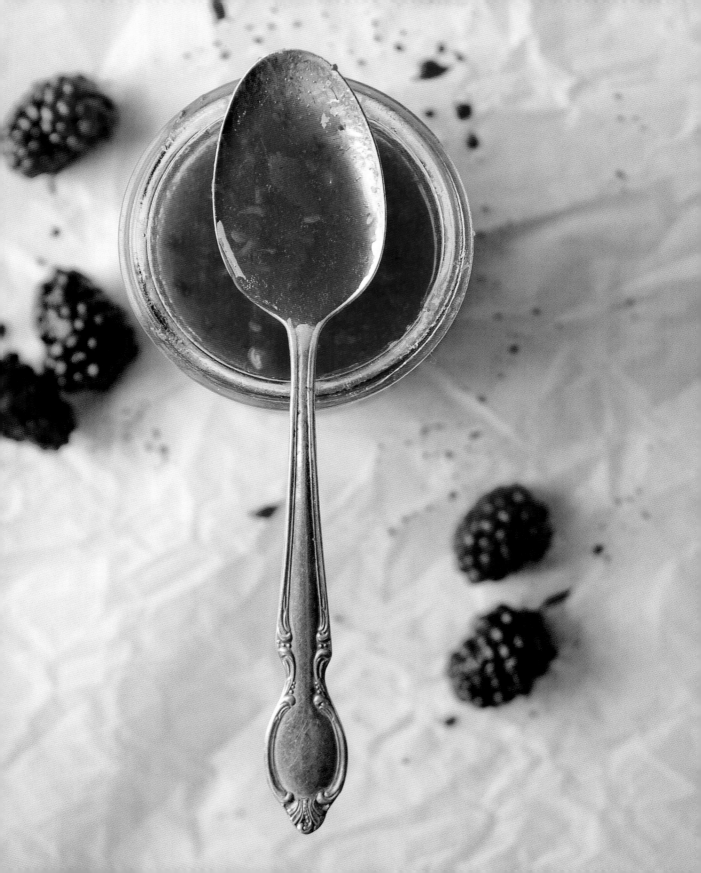

BERRY JAM FILLING

We call this jam, but it's more of a quick fruit puree or spread. For us, it's about balancing the bright, fresh flavor of perfectly ripe fruit with a bit of sweetness and acid. We usually make a small batch after a trip to the farmer's market and keep it as an essential in our fridge all week long.

MAKES 2 CUPS

2 cups fresh or frozen raspberries, strawberries, blueberries, or blackberries (or a combination)

3 tablespoons maple syrup

1 tablespoon fresh lemon juice

1. In a medium saucepan over medium heat, combine the berries, maple syrup, and lemon juice. Cook, stirring and mashing the berries, for 8 to 10 minutes, until the juices have been released and thickened. Remove the pan from the heat and allow the jam to cool.

2. Transfer the jam to a glass jar. Refrigerate until ready to use, for up to 5 days.

PROBIOTIC CREAM CHEESE FROSTING

You can't have a classic red velvet cake or a carrot cake without cream cheese frosting; that's just a fact. We developed our own take with fluffy, spreadable cashew cream. Cashews are a softer nut, and can easily be molded into a variety of treats. A probiotic capsule and lemon juice work to create the cream cheese flavor, and a blender makes it all come together into a delicious frosting.

MAKES I CUP

2¼ cups raw cashews, soaked for 1 hour, drained, and rinsed

½ cup full-fat coconut milk

½ cup maple syrup

2 tablespoons coconut oil, melted

2 teaspoons vanilla extract

1 probiotic capsule (see page 249)

1 tablespoon fresh lemon juice

½ teaspoon Himalayan pink salt

In a blender, combine 2 cups of the cashews, coconut milk, maple syrup, coconut oil, vanilla, the contents of the probiotic capsule, lemon juice, and salt. Blend until creamy. If the frosting is too thin, blend the remaining soaked cashews until smooth. Refrigerate until ready to use; the frosting will keep in a sealed container for up to 3 days.

PINK ROSE BUTTERCREAM

Rose is one of our favorite flavors to fold into our recipes. It adds a lovely delicate note, especially when paired with nuts.

MAKES 1 CUP

½ cup coconut butter

½ cup full-fat coconut milk

2 teaspoons fresh lemon juice

2 tablespoons maple syrup

2 teaspoons rose water

2 tablespoons beet juice, or as needed

In a medium saucepan over low heat, whisk together the coconut butter, coconut milk, lemon juice, and maple syrup. The frosting should be smooth, but not runny. If you find it's too runny, add a bit more coconut butter. Stir in the rose water and beet juice. If you would like the frosting to be more pink, add more beet juice.

MILK CHOCOLATE FROSTING

Creamy milk chocolate frosting is a must-have recipe. This is the frosting that ends up on kids' faces, that gets spoonfuls stolen while you're trying to whip up a batch, that you can spread on toast if you're in a "cake for breakfast" kind of mood. You can make it sweeter or milkier by adding a few more tablespoons of maple syrup or coconut milk.

MAKES 1 CUP

4 ounces 100% cacao unsweetened baking chocolate, broken into chunks

¼ cup coconut oil, solid

⅓ cup maple syrup

1 tablespoon vanilla extract

1/2 cup almond butter, store-bought or homemade (page 38)

1/2 cup full-fat coconut milk, plus more as needed

1. Melt the chocolate and coconut oil in a double boiler over medium heat, stirring constantly (see Note, page 48). Remove from the heat when melted. Add the maple syrup and vanilla and stir to incorporate. Cool to room temperature; it should still be liquid, not solid.

2. Transfer the mixture to a medium bowl and with an electric mixer beat in the almond butter until a thick, whippy frosting is formed. Add the coconut milk and continue beating until smooth.

3. For more of a sauce, use the frosting at this state. For a sturdy frosting suitable for building cakes, put the frosting in the fridge to set for at least 2 hours. Whip again until spreadable and fluffy, adding coconut milk if you need to smooth it out further. Refrigerate in a sealed container for up to 2 weeks.

COCONUT BUTTERCREAM

This is one of our staple frostings at Sweet Laurel, and we love how simple it is to make. Coconut butter is the key ingredient. It is beautiful as a natural white frosting; however, we frequently color it with one of our natural and food-based colorings (check out the variations). The best part is how smoothly it can spread—almost like fondant. This versatile frosting is incredibly fun to play with. It is the frosting used in all of the decor techniques on pages 245 to 248.

MAKES 2 CUPS

2 cups coconut butter or coconut manna

¼ cup raw honey

½ cup full-fat coconut milk or almond milk

1 teaspoon vanilla extract

Place all the ingredients in a medium saucepan over very low heat. Gently whisk until the mixture is thick and creamy. If it's a little too creamy, add a bit more coconut milk. The buttercream variations work best, at room temperature, when used immediately after making the frosting and finishing your baked goods. If you need to make it ahead, refrigerate the buttercream for up to 4 days, then allow it to come to room temperature outside of the refrigerator before using as an icing or frosting.

DEEP BLUE GREEN

Once you remove the pan from the heat, add 1 teaspoon spirulina powder and whisk until combined.

LIGHT GREEN

Once you remove the pan from the heat, add 1 teaspoon matcha powder and whisk. Be sure to work out all the lumps.

YELLOW

Once you remove the pan from the heat, add ½ teaspoon turmeric powder and whisk.

PINK

Once you remove the pan from the heat, add 2 tablespoons beet juice and whisk.

STRAWBERRY BUTTERCREAM

Once you remove the pan from the heat, add ¼ cup mashed strawberries and whisk. Stir well to diminish lumps. For a perfectly smooth frosting, puree the strawberries before adding.

OMBRÉ FROSTING

Divide the white buttercream frosting evenly among four small bowls. Stir 3 tablespoons beet juice into the first bowl, 2 tablespoons into the second bowl, and 1 tablespoon into the third bowl. Leave the remaining bowl of frosting white. This method works with any of the above colorings.

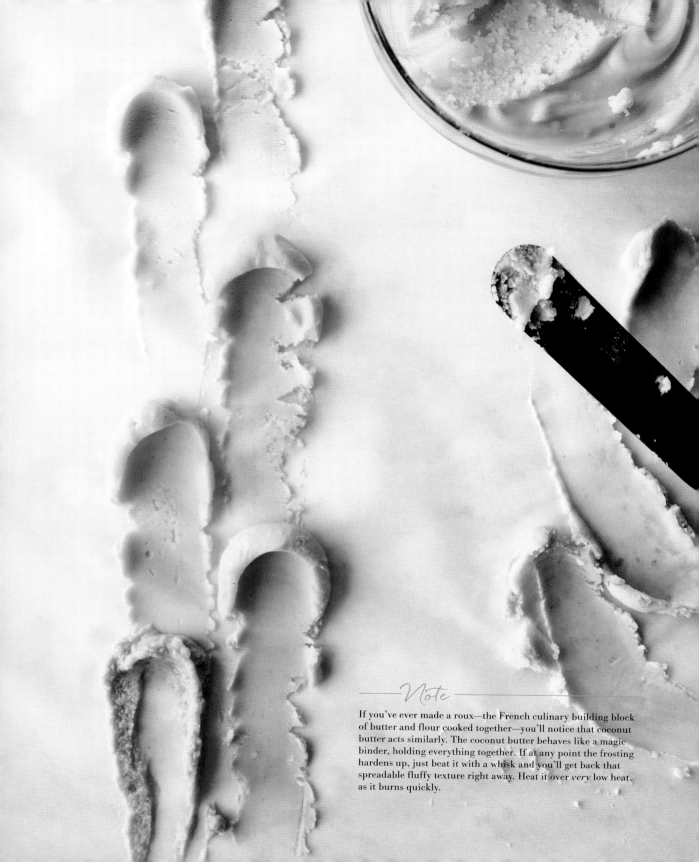

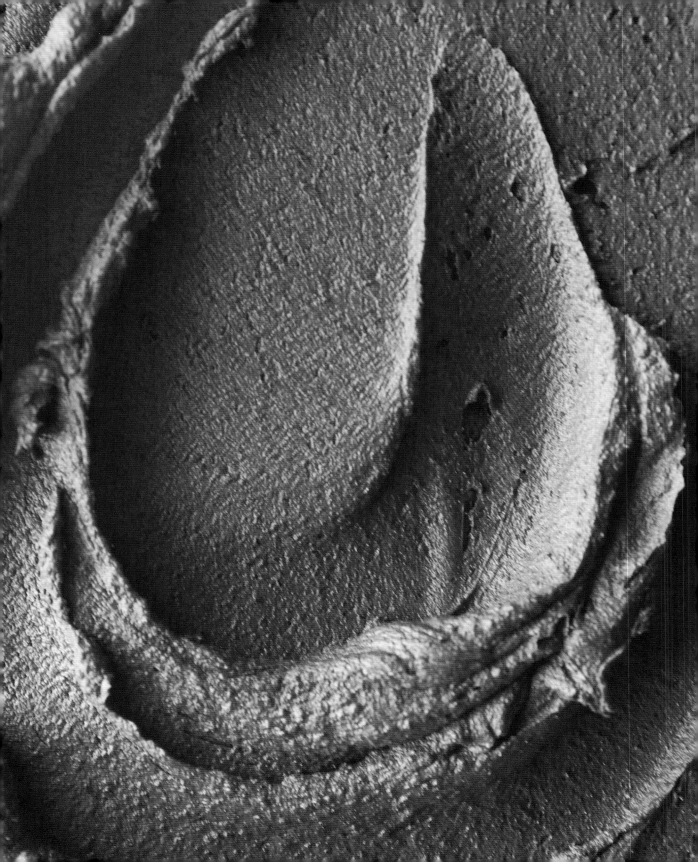

DARK CHOCOLATE FUDGE FROSTING

Herein lies the glue holding together The Chocolate Cake That Changed Everything (page 167). This frosting is delicious and decadent. It's a *dark* dark chocolate frosting. If you're not a dark chocolate fiend like us, we encourage you to add an extra 2 tablespoons of maple syrup to your batch plus a little extra coconut cream to sweeten it up.

MAKES 1 CUP

4 ounces 100% cacao unsweetened baking chocolate, roughly chopped

¼ cup coconut oil, solid

¼ cup maple syrup

½ cup almond butter, store-bought or homemade (page 38)

¼ cup almond milk or full-fat coconut milk, or as needed

1. In a small heavy saucepan over medium heat, melt the chocolate and coconut oil, stirring constantly. Remove the pan from the heat. Slowly add the maple syrup and stir to incorporate. Allow to cool completely.

2. Transfer the chocolate mixture to a medium bowl and, using an electric mixer, beat in the almond butter until a thick frosting forms. Add the almond milk and stir with a spatula until smooth.

3. For a creamy, almost pourable frosting, use immediately; for a fluffy frosting, refrigerate for at least 8 hours, then bring to room temperature and beat with an electric mixer until spreadable. Refrigerate in a sealed container for up to 2 weeks.

MEXICAN HOT CHOCOLATE GANACHE

This frosting is dangerous. Like, hide-your-spoons dangerous. The spice and cinnamon emphasize the rich cacao flavors and add a wonderful depth. We lightened up the chocolate with a little extra coconut milk to get more of a milk chocolate flavor, which is perfect with the subtle heat.

MAKES 1 CUP

4 ounces 100% cacao unsweetened baking chocolate, roughly chopped

¼ cup coconut oil, solid

¼ cup maple syrup

½ cup almond butter, store-bought or homemade (page 38)

¼ cup almond milk or full-fat coconut milk, or as needed

¼ teaspoon cayenne pepper, plus more for dusting

1 teaspoon ground cinnamon, plus more for dusting

1. In a small heavy saucepan over medium heat, melt the cacao and coconut oil, stirring constantly. Remove the pan from the heat. Slowly add the maple syrup and stir to incorporate. Allow to cool completely.

2. Transfer the cacao mixture to a medium bowl and, with an electric mixer, beat in the almond butter until a thick frosting forms. Add the almond milk, and stir with a spatula until smooth. Gently fold in the cayenne and cinnamon.

3. For a creamy, almost pourable frosting, use immediately; for a fluffy frosting, refrigerate for at least 8 hours, then bring to room temperature and beat until spreadable. Refrigerate in a sealed container for up to 2 weeks.

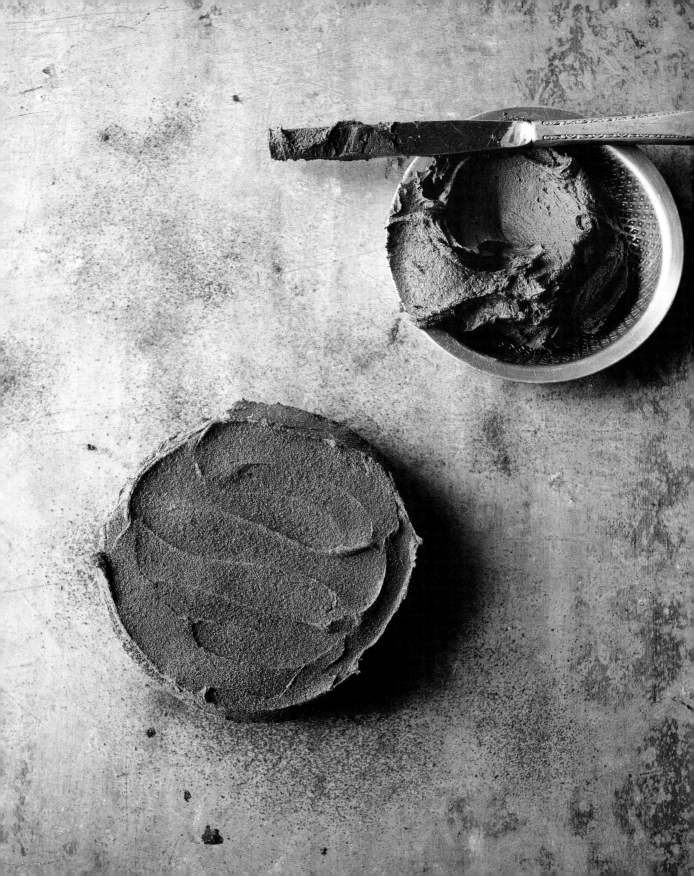

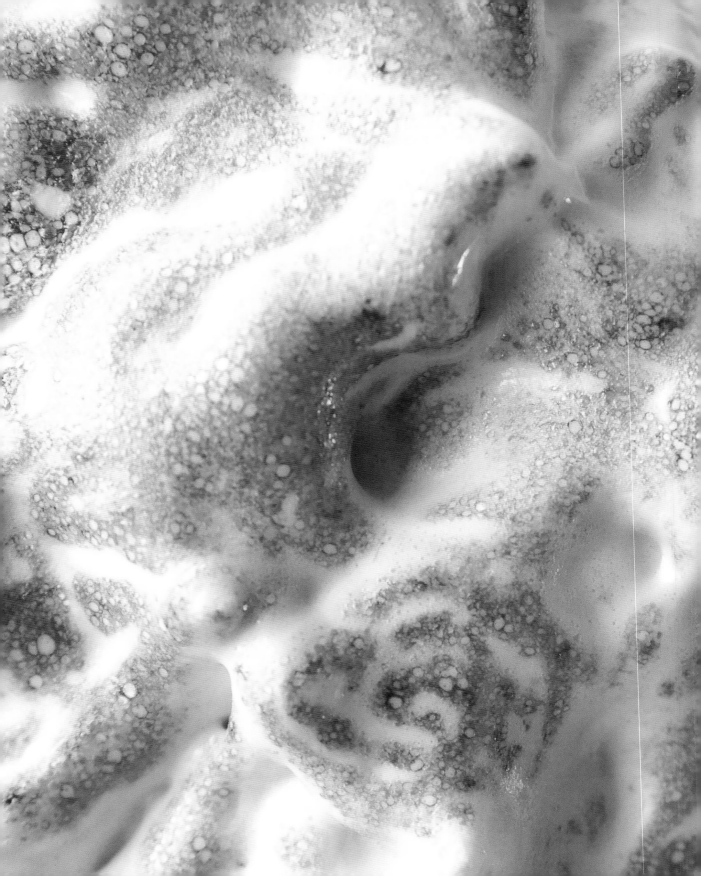

MARSHMALLOW FROSTING

COCONUT PECAN FROSTING

Marshmallow frosting is underused in the baking world, and we don't understand why. It's sweet and fluffy, and you can torch it! We love spreading this on top of citrus flavors, like on a lemon pie or grapefruit curd, where the acid cuts through the fluffy sweetness of the marshmallow, or keeping it classic and combining it with dark chocolate. The fabulous thing about the maple syrup is that it caramelizes just like cane sugar, so it torches beautifully.

Hide your spoons, because you will find yourself stealing bites of this decadent, delicious frosting until there is nothing left. We created this rich frosting for our German Chocolate Cake (page 196), but it's also perfect with our Pumpkin Spice Latte Cake (page 172) or even our Dark Horse Carrot Cake (page 171).

MAKES 4 TO 5 CUPS

3 tablespoons gelatin

1 cup maple syrup

1 teaspoon vanilla extract

MAKES 3½ CUPS

1 cup full-fat coconut milk

1 cup maple syrup

½ cup coconut oil, melted

3 large egg yolks, lightly beaten

⅛ teaspoon

Himalayan pink salt

1½ teaspoons vanilla extract

1⅓ cups unsweetened shredded coconut

1 cup pecans, lightly toasted and finely chopped

1. Pour ½ cup water into the bowl of a stand mixer fitted with the whisk attachment and sprinkle the gelatin on top to soften. Gently stir to combine.

2. In a medium saucepan over medium heat, combine ½ cup water, the maple syrup, and vanilla. Bring the mixture to a simmer, and use a candy thermometer to monitor the temperature until it reaches 240°F. Remove from the heat and be ready to immediately add it to the gelatin and water.

3. With the mixer on medium-high, blend the gelatin and water. Slowly pour in the syrup mixture and continue to beat for about 10 minutes, until the steam disappears and soft marshmallow peaks form. Use the marshmallow frosting immediately, as the longer it sits, the more it will set. If the frosting sets too quickly, put the bowl over some hot water to loosen it up and beat on low or, in a pinch, pour the set frosting into a glass bowl and microwave for 30 seconds on low.

1. In a medium saucepan, combine the coconut milk, maple syrup, coconut oil, egg yolks, and salt. Cook over medium heat, stirring constantly, until the mixture is bubbly and thickened or reaches 170°F on a candy thermometer, about 20 minutes. Remove from the heat and add the vanilla.

2. Stir in the coconut and pecans. Continue stirring until cooled and thick enough to spread, about 1 hour. The frosting will keep in a sealed container in the fridge for up to a week.

Note

This frosting is especially versatile—you can swap the pecans with any nut, or add delicious flavorings like spices or citrus zest.

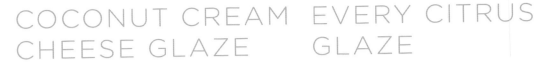

COCONUT CREAM CHEESE GLAZE

EVERY CITRUS GLAZE

Be prepared to fall in love—this sweet and tart coconut glaze will soon find its way onto all of your favorite buns, rolls, and breads. The texture is creamy and perfectly spreadable, and the glaze is super simple to put together.

If you love baking (and we assume you do!), this is one of those recipes you'll want to have at the ready. It goes equally well on doughnuts and teacakes, scones and cookies . . . you could drizzle it over almost anything. It's super versatile and one of our favorites.

MAKES I CUP

MAKES ½ CUP

½ cup coconut butter, also known as coconut manna, plus more as needed

2 tablespoons maple syrup

1 teaspoon vanilla extract

½ cup coconut yogurt, store-bought or homemade (page 40), plus more as needed

¼ cup coconut butter, plus more as needed

2 teaspoons maple syrup or raw honey

½ teaspoon fresh lemon juice

¼ teaspoon vanilla extract

¼ cup full-fat coconut milk or almond milk, plus more as needed

Grated zest of 1 lemon

In a small saucepan, combine the coconut butter, maple syrup, vanilla, and coconut yogurt over very low heat. Whisk until smooth, about 5 minutes. If the icing is too thick, add a little more yogurt. If it's too runny, add more coconut butter. Store in a sealed container in the fridge for up to a week, reheating and stirring to loosen.

1. Combine the coconut butter, maple syrup, lemon juice, vanilla, and coconut milk in a medium saucepan over very low heat and stir constantly for about 5 minutes, until the mixture is smooth and slightly thickened.

2. Remove the pan from the heat and allow to cool to room temperature, then stir in the lemon zest. If you'd like your icing thinner, add more coconut milk; for a thicker glaze, add more coconut butter. Use the glaze immediately, or refrigerate for up to 4 days and reheat over low heat before using.

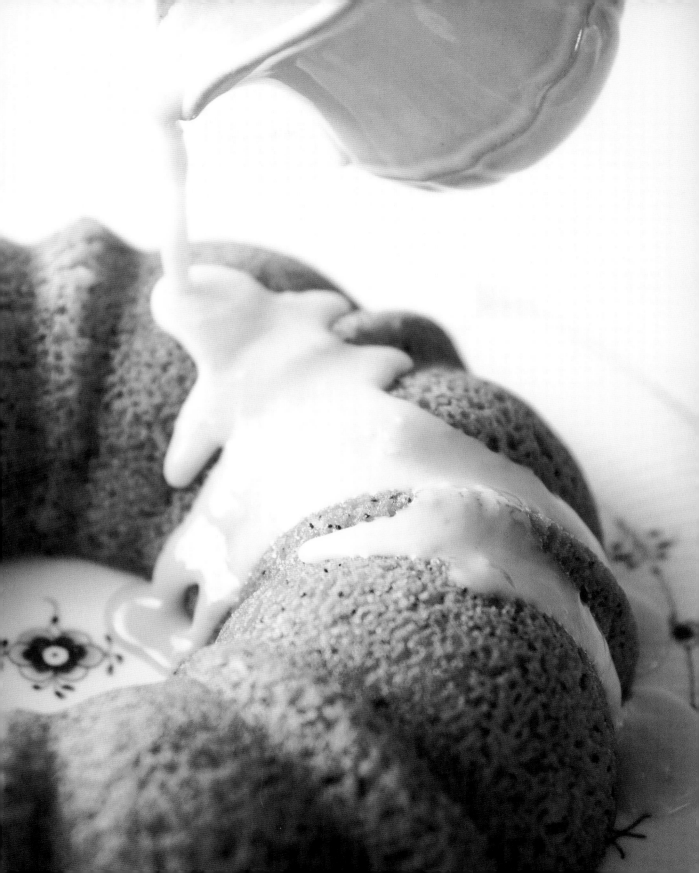

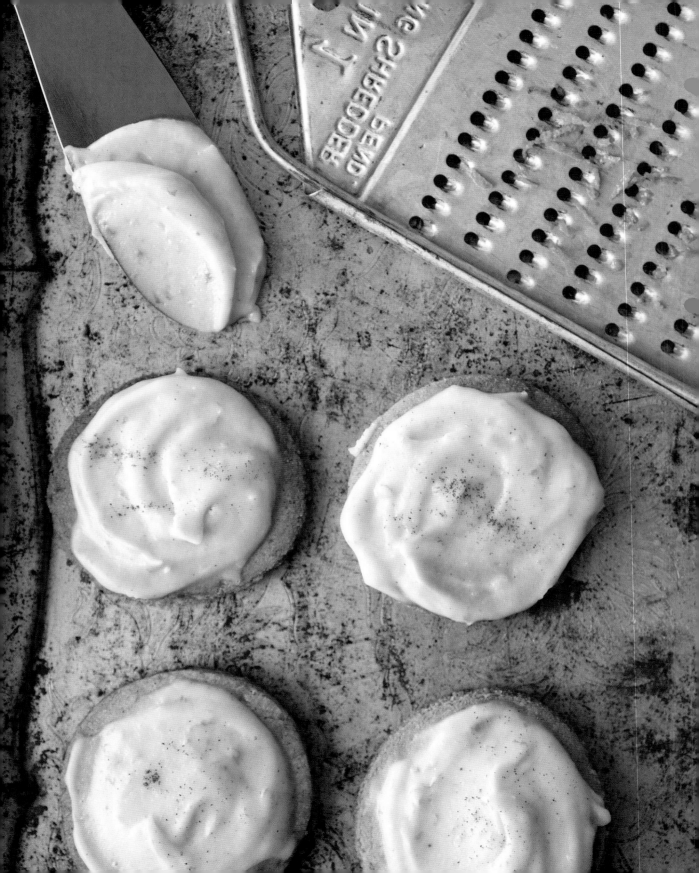

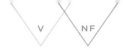

ORANGE COCONUT GLAZE

Fresh, bright, and perfectly suited to any citrus fruit, this orange glaze is a fabulous addition to your repertoire. We spread it on cookies and loaves, or thin it out and drizzle it on Bundt cakes. It's simply so, so good.

MAKES 1 CUP

½ cup coconut butter, plus more as needed

2 tablespoons maple syrup

1 teaspoon vanilla extract

1 tablespoon grated orange zest

¼ cup full-fat coconut milk, plus more as needed

¼ cup fresh orange juice

In a small saucepan, combine the coconut butter, maple syrup, vanilla, zest, coconut milk, and orange juice over very low heat. Whisk until smooth, about 5 minutes. If the icing is too thick, add a little more coconut milk. If it's too runny, add more coconut butter. Store in a sealed container in the fridge for up to a week.

CANDIED GINGER SYRUP

We love this simple candied ginger syrup drizzled on cakes, mixed into whipped cream, added to hot water for a delicious tea, or even just eaten with a spoon out of the jar.

MAKES 2 CUPS GINGER IN SYRUP

8 ounces fresh ginger

1¼ cups maple syrup

1. Peel the ginger and slice it about ⅛ inch thick. Using a mandoline is the easiest way to do this.

2. Bring the ginger and 2 cups water to a boil in a medium pot over high heat. Reduce the heat to medium low and simmer, covered, for 30 minutes, then uncover and continue to simmer for another 10 to 15 minutes, until tender.

3. Drain all but ½ cup water from the pan and add the maple syrup. Simmer for another 30 minutes, until the syrup has thickened and the ginger is translucent. Remove from the heat. Store in a sealed container in the fridge for up to 3 weeks.

—— *Note* ——

This recipe doesn't create crystalized ginger like you'll see in the candy shop, but rather, sweet, tender ginger chunks and delicious ginger syrup. Both elements add lovely spice and brightness to any recipe, and they last for weeks in the fridge.

LEMON SPREAD

Our spin on lemon curd, this lemon spread is perfect for your next tea and scones affair. When Laurel was growing up, her mother took her to afternoon tea on special occasions, where she taught her proper respect for lemon curd and clotted cream. Laurel now throws tea parties of her own, without the refined sugar and dairy, and this lemon spread is always served as an accompaniment. Pair it with our Coconut Whipped Cream (page 30) and Mother's Scones (page 46), and your tea party will be complete!

MAKES 1 CUP

3 large eggs

2 tablespoons grated lemon zest

⅓ cup maple syrup

½ cup fresh lemon juice

¼ cup plus 2 tablespoons coconut oil, melted

1. In a medium bowl, whisk together the eggs, lemon zest, and maple syrup. In a small bowl, stir together the lemon juice and coconut oil.

2. Pour the egg mixture into a medium saucepan and cook over low heat, whisking constantly, until it begins to thicken, 10 to 15 minutes. Do not overcook, as the eggs will become lumpy. Slowly stir in the lemon juice and coconut oil and cook, constantly whisking, until the mixture thickens further, another 10 to 15 minutes. If you're not sure if it's thick enough, stop stirring for a few seconds and see if large, slow bubbles form on the surface. It should have the texture of loose pudding. Do not boil.

3. Remove the pan from the heat and pour the mixture through a fine-mesh sieve into a glass jar. Let cool, then seal and refrigerate until ready to use, up to 1 week.

Notes

Because you want this spread to be a pretty, bright yellow, be sure to use A-grade maple syrup that is light in color.

This recipe is quite tart, and is meant to pair with sweet baked goods. But if you prefer a sweeter lemon spread, feel free to add an extra tablespoon of maple syrup.

This recipe is delicious when made with lime or grapefruit juice and zest as well!

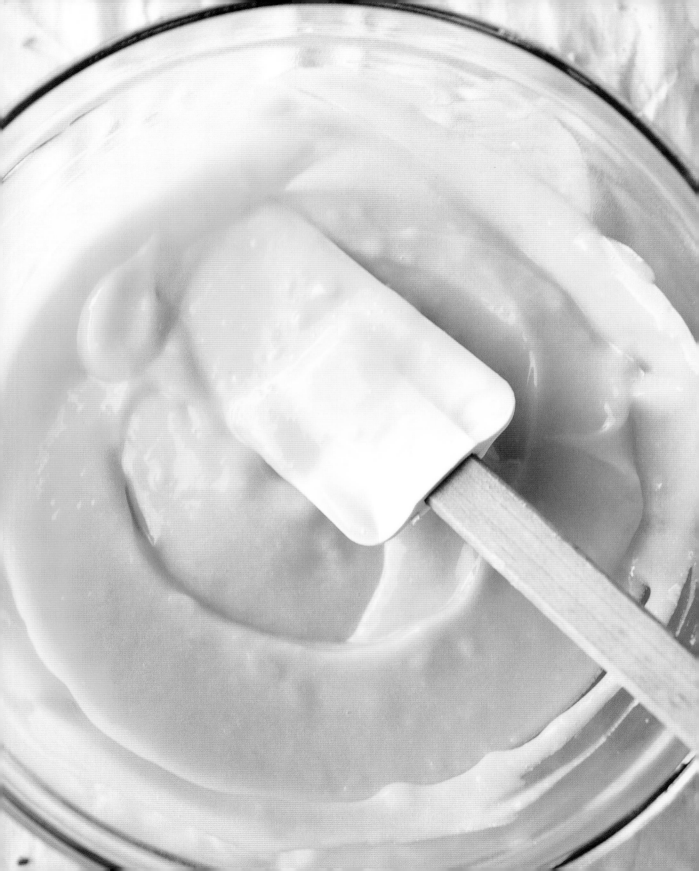

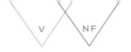

PALEO SPRINKLES

When Claire was young, her mother would make her pixie bread: white bread and butter with sprinkles on top. This was the meal of choice for her dolls. There's something about the bright speckles of color in sprinkles that simply puts smiles on our faces and makes us feel like kids again. But if you're trying to maintain a clean diet, or are staying away from refined sugar, conventional sprinkles are a no-go. Luckily, these are easy to make and we love the subtle, elegant color palette you get from natural dyes.

MAKES 2 CUPS

1 cup cacao butter or cocoa butter, roughly chopped (see Notes)

1 cup coconut milk powder (see Notes)

1 teaspoon vanilla extract

Pinch of Himalayan pink salt

2 tablespoons raw honey

Coloring (see below)

1. Line a rimmed baking sheet with parchment paper.

2. In a heavy medium saucepan, melt the cacao butter over low heat, stirring constantly. Whisk in the coconut milk powder, vanilla, and salt and stir until completely smooth. Remove from the heat and allow to cool for about 10 minutes.

3. Slowly stir in the honey and the coloring of your choice.

4. There are two options for creating sprinkles. For more rustic sprinkles, pour the mixture into the prepared pan and refrigerate until hardened. Using a sharp knife, chop into very small, sprinkle-like pieces. For more conventional sprinkles, put the mixture into a pastry bag with a #4 pastry tip. Squeeze out lines across the baking sheet, careful not to overlap, and then put the baking sheet in the fridge until the sprinkles set, about 1 hour. Chop the lines into ¼-inch pieces. Store in a sealed container for up to 2 months.

PINK SPRINKLES

When you add the honey, also add 2 tablespoons beet juice.

YELLOW SPRINKLES

When you add the honey, also add ½ teaspoon turmeric powder.

GREEN SPRINKLES

When you add the honey, also add 1 teaspoon matcha powder.

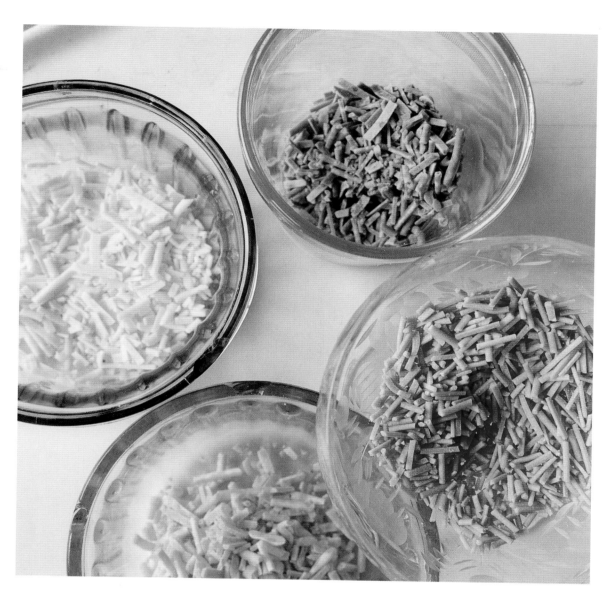

Notes

Cacao butter (which is a raw food) or cocoa butter (which is roasted) is the main ingredient in white chocolate, so you might experience a lot of the same frustrations working with it. The most important thing is temperature—always work over a low heat. Also, be sure your pan is completely dry (moisture will make the cacao butter seize up). If it starts to coagulate, it got too hot and is unsalvageable. This is a massive bummer, but really easy to do, so stay vigilant.

Coconut milk powder is simply dehydrated coconut milk mixed with a small amount of tapioca starch. The brand we like is Z Natural Foods Organic Coconut Milk Powder. We use it in our sprinkles, and Laurel likes to use it to make morning mochas and cups of hot cocoa. When mixed with water, it creates an instant coconut milk stand-in.

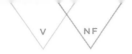

TWO-INGREDIENT ICE CREAM

It's crazy how two ingredients can create something so delicious, but don't under-estimate the power of coconut cream and honey. This recipe is as simple as it gets, but feel free to add your favorite mix-ins to personalize the flavor and texture. And of course, have some Vegan Caramel (page 40) handy for liberal drizzling. We like to let this ice cream sit on the counter for 15 minutes for easier scooping.

MAKES 1 PINT

2 cups coconut cream (about 2 to 3 cans of full-fat coconut milk), at room temperature

¼ cup raw honey, plus more for serving

In a large bowl, whisk together the coconut cream and honey. Cover the bowl with plastic wrap and refrigerate for at least 2 hours, or until thoroughly cold. Freeze the mixture in your ice cream maker according to the manufacturer's instructions. Serve drizzled with honey.

___ *Note* ___

Be sure the ice cream is thoroughly chilled before putting it in the ice cream maker. Coconut cream has a habit of hardening when frozen, and letting the ice cream almost fully set in the ice cream maker creates finer and smoother ice crystals.

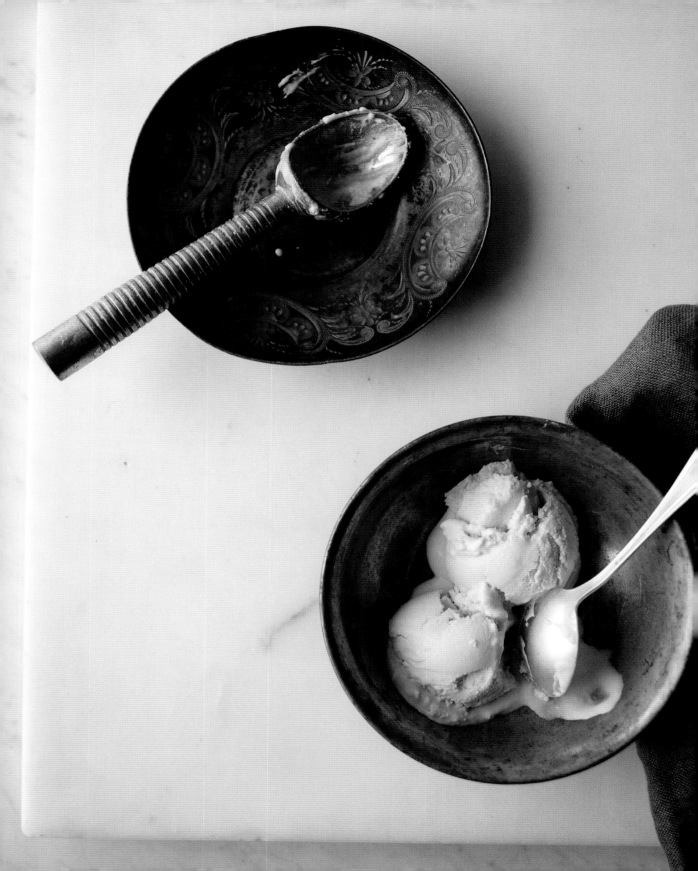

CREAMY DAIRY-FREE ICE CREAM

For a creamy, classic ice cream texture, this recipe is perfect. The egg yolks add richness and fat, creating a finer, more scoopable ice cream than the preceding two-ingredient vegan option. This is our basic vanilla recipe, but by mixing and matching flavors like a frozen dessert alchemist, you can create scoops that are entirely customized for your palate.

MAKES 1 QUART

1 cup full-fat coconut milk

2 cups coconut cream

¾ cup honey

Pinch of Himalayan pink salt

5 large egg yolks

1 teaspoon vanilla extract

1. In a medium saucepan over medium heat, warm the coconut milk, 1 cup of the coconut cream, the honey, and salt, stirring until blended. Pour the remaining 1 cup coconut cream into a large bowl and set a fine-mesh sieve on top.

2. Beat the egg yolks in a medium bowl, then slowly pour the warmed coconut mixture into the egg yolks, whisking constantly. Transfer the entire mixture back into the saucepan and stir constantly over medium heat, being sure to scrape the bottom of the pan as you stir. Remove the custard from the heat when it thickens and coats the back of a spoon, about 10 minutes.

3. Set up an ice bath by filling another large bowl with water and ice. Pour the custard through the sieve and stir it into the coconut cream. Mix in the vanilla, set the bowl with the cream mixture over the ice bath, and stir until cool.

4. Chill the mixture in the refrigerator for about an hour, then freeze in an ice cream maker according to the manufacturer's instructions. Store in a sealed container in the freezer for at least 2 hours to set.

STRAWBERRY ICE CREAM

Strawberry completes the triumvirate of classic ice cream flavors—vanilla and chocolate being the other two. And for some reason, it seems to get overlooked. But we love the simple, bright flavor of fresh strawberries mixed into our creamy coconut ice cream base. It's not too sweet and pairs beautifully with our fruit-based cakes and baked treats. The key is a touch of lemon, to keep the strawberries a pretty bright red and add a hint of acid.

MAKES 1 QUART

1 cup full-fat coconut milk

2 cups coconut cream

¾ cup honey

Pinch of Himalayan pink salt

¾ cup mashed strawberries

1 tablespoon fresh lemon juice

5 large egg yolks

1 teaspoon vanilla extract

1. In a medium saucepan over medium heat, warm the coconut milk, 1 cup of the coconut cream, the honey, and salt until heated through. Pour the remaining 1 cup coconut cream into a large bowl and set a fine-mesh sieve on top.

2. Combine the mashed strawberries and lemon juice and set aside.

3. Beat the egg yolks in a medium bowl and slowly pour the warmed coconut mixture into the egg yolks, whisking constantly. Transfer the entire mixture back into the saucepan and stir constantly over medium heat, being sure to scrape the bottom of the pan as you stir. Remove the custard from the heat when it thickens and coats the back of a spoon, about 10 minutes.

4. Set up an ice bath by filling another large bowl with water and ice. Pour the custard through the sieve and stir it into the coconut cream. Mix in the vanilla, set the bowl with the cream mixture over the ice bath, and stir until cool.

5. Chill the mixture in the refrigerator for about an hour, then freeze in your ice cream maker according to the manufacturer's instructions. Halfway through the freezing process, when the ice cream looks like soft serve, add the mashed strawberries. Continue freezing. Store in a sealed container in the freezer for at least 2 hours to set.

DAIRY-FREE MINT ICE CREAM

This flavor combination is our absolute favorite, so much so that we included it in our Mint Chocolate Chip Ice Cream Cake (page 191). The fresh mint juice gives it a bright, just-plucked-from-the-garden flavor that pairs deliciously with our vegan chocolate chips.

MAKES 1 QUART

1 cup full-fat coconut milk

2 cups coconut cream

¾ cup honey

Pinch of Himalayan pink salt

5 large egg yolks

1 teaspoon vanilla extract

FOR THE MINT JUICE

1 bunch fresh mint

2 tablespoons full-fat coconut milk

1 cup vegan chocolate chips, store-bought or homemade (page 42)

1. In a medium saucepan over medium heat, warm the coconut milk, 1 cup of the coconut cream, the honey, and salt, stirring until blended. Pour the remaining 1 cup coconut cream into a large bowl and set a fine-mesh sieve on top.

2. Beat the egg yolks in a medium bowl, then slowly pour the warmed coconut mixture into the egg yolks, whisking constantly. Transfer the entire mixture back into the saucepan and stir constantly over medium heat, being sure to scrape the bottom of the pan as you stir. Remove the custard from the heat when it thickens and coats the back of a spoon, about 10 minutes.

3. Set up an ice bath by filling another large bowl with water and ice. Pour the custard through the sieve and stir it into the coconut cream. Mix in the vanilla, set the bowl with the cream mixture over the ice bath, and stir until cool. Chill the mixture thoroughly in the refrigerator.

4. **MAKE THE MINT JUICE:** Combine the mint, coconut milk, and 2 tablespoons water in a blender and pulse until completely pureed.

5. Pour the mint juice through a nut-milk bag to strain. Then pour the ice cream custard and the mint juice into an ice cream maker and freeze according to the manufacturer's instructions. Slowly add the chocolate chips while the ice cream processes. Store in a sealed container in the freezer for at least 2 hours to set.

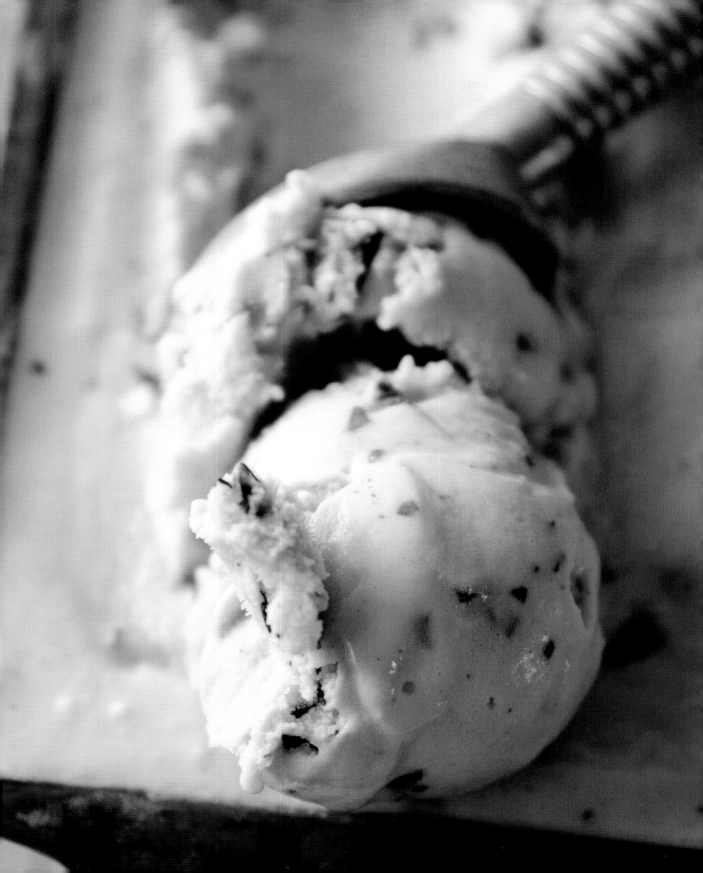

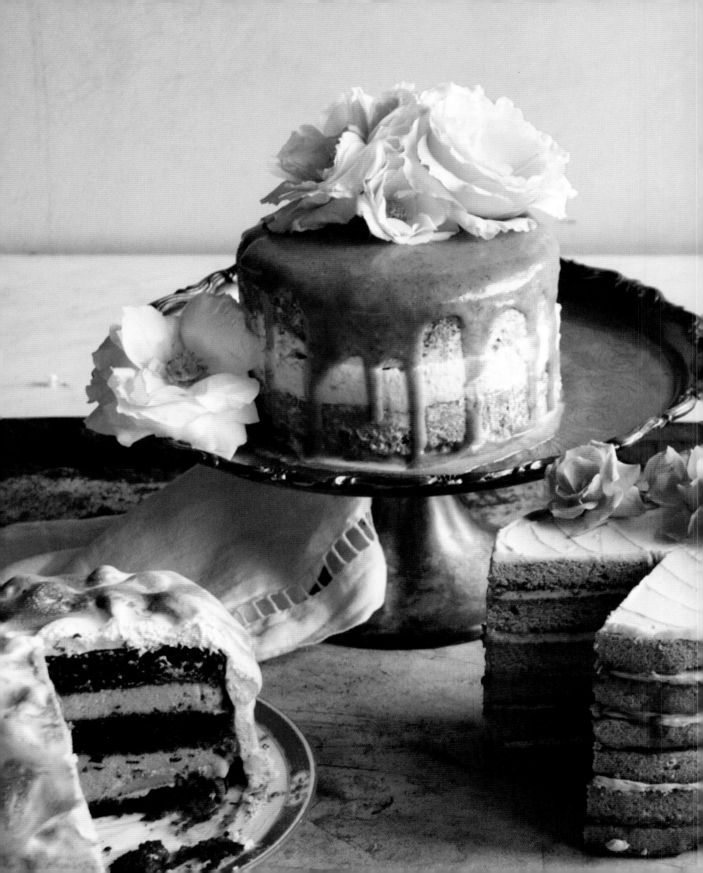

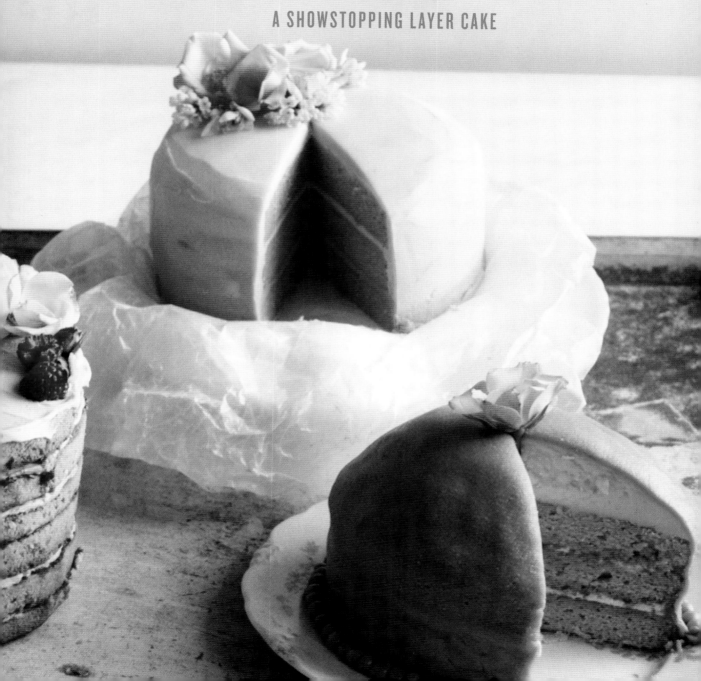

The GRAND FINALE

HOW TO CREATE AND DECORATE
A SHOWSTOPPING LAYER CAKE

The most important thing about any dessert is how it tastes: that combination of sweetness and beautiful textures that begs a second bite. Taste is how we got customers, but it was the visual component that made Sweet Laurel a national brand. Our look is unfussy, modern, and feminine, and here's the secret—it's really easy. Neither of us was very good at making flowers out of buttercream, or piping "Happy Birthday" across a cake. We can't roll out a decent fondant and we can't make sugar roses. But sexy drips of caramel and some gorgeous flowers? Done and done!

Our aversion to overly ambitious frosting art ended up being a blessing in disguise. We turned toward a more minimalist, loose aesthetic, letting the ingredients speak for themselves. We'd add fresh fruit, nuts, or organic flowers if we wanted a more striking effect. Soon, how our cakes looked became as popular as how our cakes tasted. At workshops, guests would clamor for lessons on how to create the "Sweet Laurel" look. What's so funny is how simple it actually is. We understand that cake decorating can be intimidating. You've just put in all this effort, and now you have to become a frosting architect of sorts. Trust us, you'll be whipping up glorious centerpiece cakes of your own in no time.

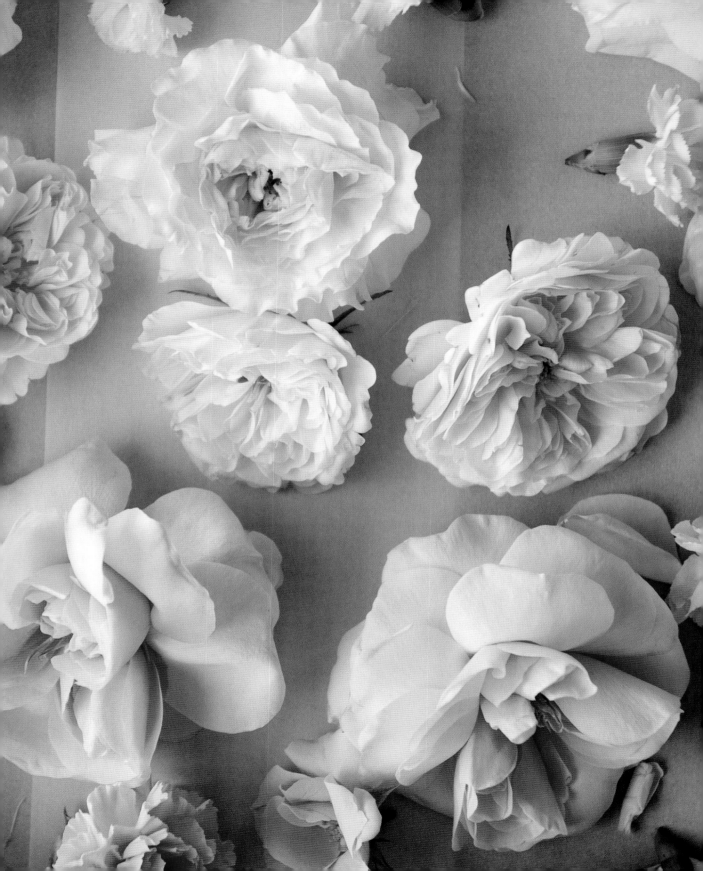

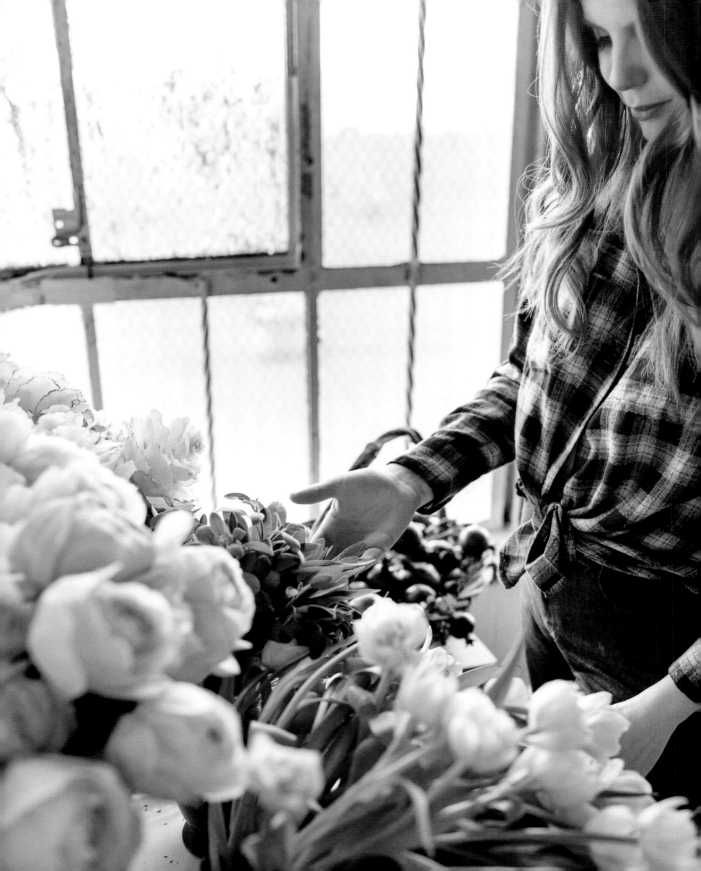

HOW TO BUILD A NAKED CAKE

The signature look for a Sweet Laurel cake is a naked cake. Exposed on the sides, jam or caramel or whatever delicious ingredient we're featuring dripping down the sides, with coconut cream or frosting holding everything together. If everything looks too tidy, it can look like a forgotten cake, stiff and begging for adornment. If it's too messy, it looks like a *really* forgotten cake, as in, forgotten in the sun for too long. There's a balance that needs to be struck for a cake that is perfectly romantic and unfussy, but still delicious and appealing looking.

You'll notice that some of our cakes call for being sliced into thin layers and some we leave whole. This is entirely up to personal preference. Turning a 3-layer cake into 6 thin layers creates a taller, more substantial-looking cake, and also gives us a higher cake-to-frosting ratio. Laurel is more about cake with a little bit of frosting, and Claire is a frosting nut, so you can guess who is decorating which cake based on the frosting amount alone.

Start with a completely cool cake. If your cake is at all warm, it will melt the frosting and cause everything to slide around. Be patient!

If you're slicing your cake in half, you will need:

1. A sharp knife (we use a serrated bread knife)
2. A cake platter or lazy susan
3. Toothpicks, optional

Place one layer of cake onto the cake platter or lazy susan. If you're not sure of your knife skills, stab the cake with toothpicks in a neat row, marking the halfway point of the cake layer around the circumference. It will look like spokes on a wheel. The toothpicks will serve as a guide for your knife.

When you're ready to slice, line up the knife with the center of the cake layer (or just above the toothpicks, if using) and start gently sawing the cake. With your other hand, gently turn the cake stand or lazy susan, so you can smoothly slice the cake layer in half.

Once the cake layer is halved, set aside both halves on a plate and start slicing the other layers. Don't forget to remove the toothpicks before decorating!

Now for the fun part! To decorate your cake, place one layer onto the cake platter, centered. For halved layers you will use about 3 tablespoons of filling per layer (so,

if using two fillings, 1 to 2 tablespoons of each), and for whole layers, closer to ¼ to ½ cup of filling per layer. A filling could be coconut whipped cream, jam, frosting, whatever is holding the cake together.

Spoon the appropriate amount of filling onto the center of the cake. If using two fillings, start with whichever is sturdier. Then, using an offset spatula (or if you don't have one, a butter knife will do), spread the filling just to the edge of the cake. You want the filling to gently reach to the edge as you add layers, not drip messily, so don't push the filling too far. A millimeter or two from the edge of the cake is just right. The filling should be a bit thicker toward the edge than in the center, as you spread the filling. If using two fillings, add the next one, following the same method. Add the next layer of cake. Repeat until the cake is finished except for the final layer.

For the top, expect to use more of the filling than between the other layers. Use the same method as before, but smooth the filling evenly over the top, being careful not to go over the edges. To get the Sweet Laurel "Swoop," see page 247.

At this point, you should have a finished, naked cake. If you want to create a look similar to our Tres Leches Cake (page 187), where there's a thin sweep of frosting around the cake, simply take your offset spatula and run it around the outside edge of the cake. This will create a rustic "crumb coat" look.

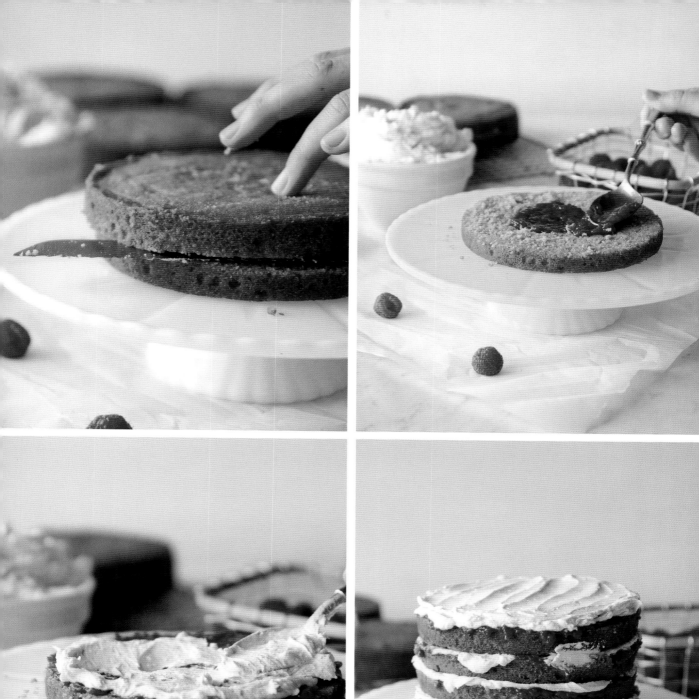

DECORATING WITH BOTANICALS

Our most popular look is the flower-topped cake, especially for weddings. We love that these cakes double as an epic centerpiece. There are a few important things to know about when decorating with botanicals:

1. SOME BOTANICALS ARE TOXIC. Meaning, poisonous. See our chart below, and be sure to check first whether the specific plant you want to decorate with is edible. For instance, if you love the look of ranunculus but know that they're toxic in concentrated doses, you could either wrap their stems in floral tape and aluminum foil, or use floral water tubes you can find at a DIY store. This way, the cut stems aren't secreting into the cake. But this is definitely a "use at your discretion" situation. As with consuming raw egg, make the choice that makes you the most comfortable.

2. BUY ORGANIC. If you can find organic flowers, use those. You don't want to decorate an edible item with something coated in pesticides. If you can't find organic, be sure to gently rinse the blooms and pat them dry right before using them. Our best source for organic flowers is the farmer's market, as a lot of the organic farmers grow flowers on their property. You can also order organic flowers online. Rose Story Farm is our favorite resource for organic roses.

Some Common Toxic Flowers

Daffodil	Lily of the valley
Foxglove	Ranunculus
Hydrangea	

Some Common Nontoxic Plants for Decorating

Chrysanthemums	Mint
Fruit blossoms (e.g., cherry blossoms, orange blossoms)	Nasturtiums
	Pansies
Jasmine	Rosemary
Lavender	Roses
Lilac	Sage
Marigolds	Violets

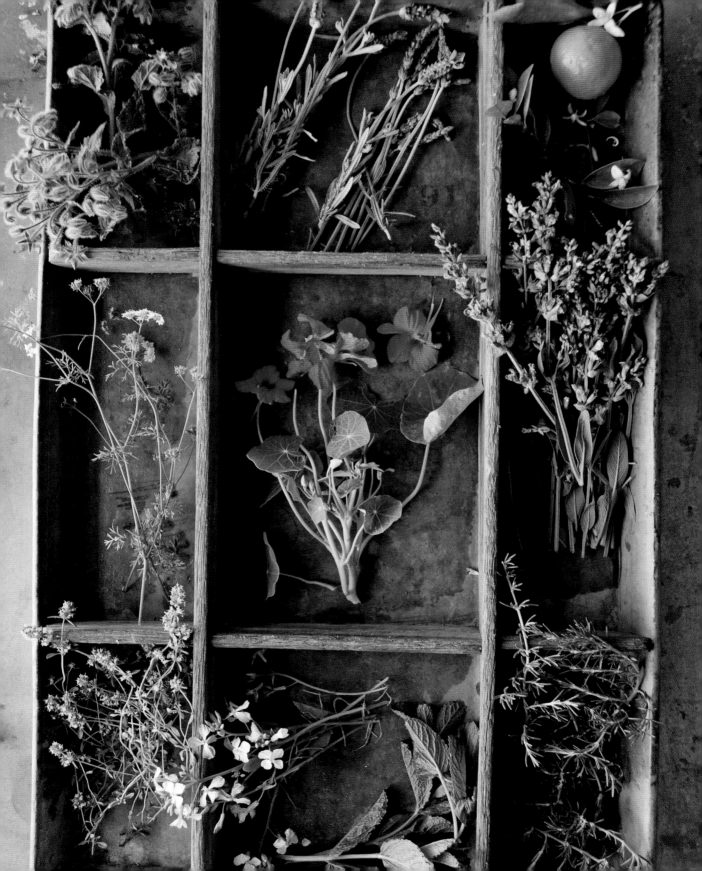

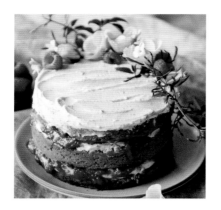

The Sweet Laurel Look

Our classic cake boasts a crescent of flowers cascading toward the edge of the cake. To get this effect, trim all of your stems down to about 1 inch so they will sit in the cake without stabbing through. Next, place three "anchor flowers" in a little group along the edge of the cake. Anchor flowers are the larger, more eye-catching flowers, like roses. We usually do a combo of a large open bloom, a slightly smaller one, and a bud. Once you've placed this group, take your greens (usually mint or rosemary for us) and put one stem emanating from each side of the anchor group, curving toward the edge of the cake. Then just lightly fill in the area along the greens with smaller, textural flowers or fruit.

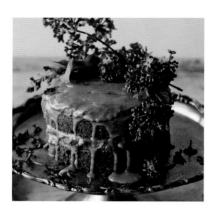

Single Flowers

When something as abundant and pretty as lilac is in season, we feel like "more is more" is the way to go. We pile on bunches of it in a curve along the cake's edge, and then press the greens into the side of the cake. You could allow the greens to poke out, but we prefer the look of greens clinging to the cake, as if they're growing out of it. This look works especially well with vine plants, like jasmine, or flowers that hang heavily, like lilac.

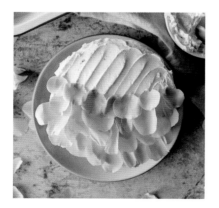

Ombré

The key to this look is finding a plant that comes in a variety of hues, or using multiple types of flowers in different grades of color. Spray roses and carnations come in a wonderful variety of colors. To get this effect, pull off all of the petals and organize them by color. Beginning with the lightest hue, create one row of petals along the bottom third of the top of the cake. Then add another row, overlapping slightly, in a slightly darker hue, above this row. Repeat until the entire cake is covered. This scale effect can be done in one color as well, and is super beautiful. We love the dynamic sweep of ombré.

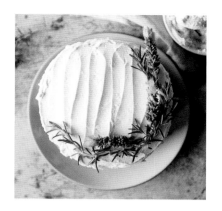

Laurel Crown

We love the look of a classic laurel crown (think Caesar). It's actually inspired by Laurel's maiden name: Laurel Czer (pronounced like Caesar), and happens to be her favorite decorating technique. The key to this look is the curve with a center intersection point. Lavender or bay leaves are great for this, as the stalks are quite pliable. Place one lavender blossom with a short stem—about an inch—on the edge of the cake, and then add another blossom facing the opposite direction, intersecting the first blossom, to create a crown shape. Keep adding blossoms to each side to get a fuller look.

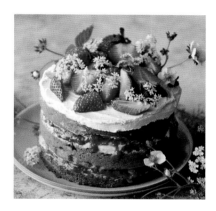

Fruit Only

You can create all of the above-described looks with fresh fruit if finding the right flowers is challenging. Berries work well, thanks to their variety and shape. The best effect comes from scouring the farmer's market for unusual or unique produce. White strawberries, gooseberries with the paper still on—these kinds of details can add so much to the decoration.

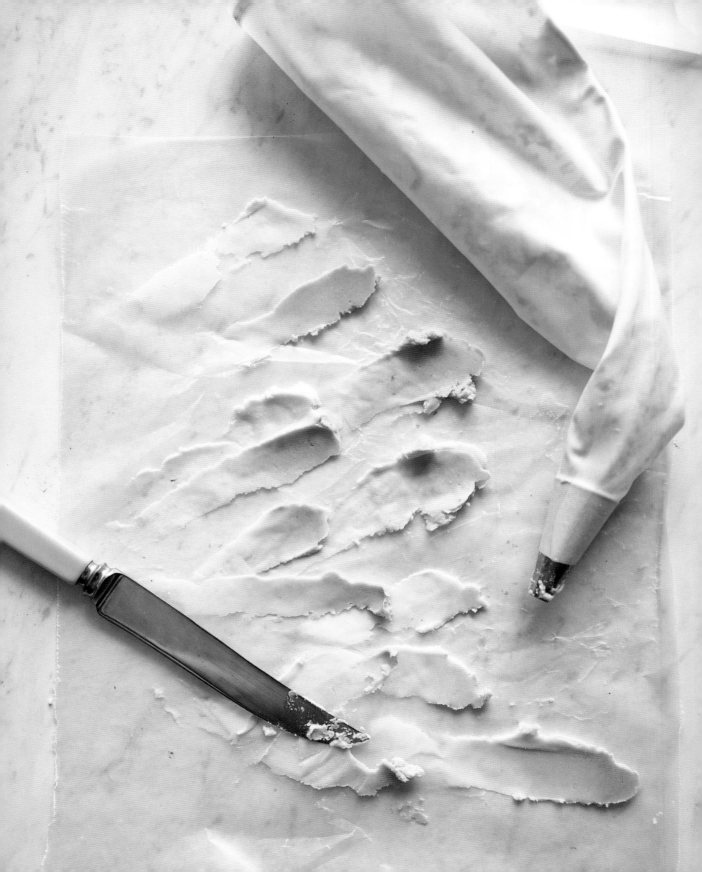

DECORATING WITH FROSTING

These techniques are super simple, and if we can do them, you certainly can, too. But first, some tips:

1. TEMPERATURE MATTERS. The ideal temperature for frosting is chilled but not quite cold. It should be a few degrees cooler than the room. If you're piping your frosting, the heat from your hands will cause it to warm and loosen, creating a messy effect. If the frosting warms in the room, it might separate and curdle a bit. The easiest fix for warm frosting is to pop it in the fridge for an hour, then beat it with an electric mixer again to reconstitute its texture.

2. CREATE A CRUMB COAT. If you're covering your entire cake in frosting and you don't want crumbs marring the surface, do a crumb coat. Just put a thin layer of frosting over the entire cake, wiping down your spatula as you go. This will keep the crumbs from traveling into the main layers of frosting as you decorate.

3. WORK OFF OF A CAKE PLATE or other elevated platform. It's just much easier than a flat plate on a counter, giving your hands space to travel.

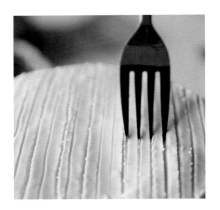

Pinstripe

Tidy rows of pinstripes are a quick and easy way to add detail to an otherwise simple cake. Frost a cake as cleanly as possible, with at least a ½-inch-thick layer all around. Take a fork, and gently move it across the top of the frosting, making stripes. Wipe the fork between passes and be careful not to press too deeply. This works best with vegan caramel, coconut buttercream, or chocolate frostings.

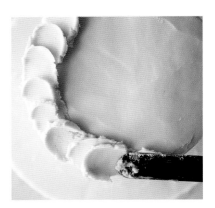

Swipes

This is the fussiest of our simple tricks, but super pretty if you can get the hang of it. It works best with coconut buttercream or chocolate frostings. Frost a cake as cleanly as possible, with at least a ¼-inch-thick layer all around. Fill the tip of an offset spatula with frosting, and gently swipe it at the base of the cake. Fill up the spatula again, and swipe about 1 inch away from the start of your first swoop, so the swoops overlap slightly, working your way up the cake. Continue in this pattern for as long as you like, until you're happy with the aesthetic.

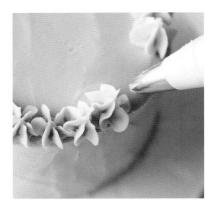

Piping

Choose a pastry tip (we like star tips best) and place it into the bottom of a pastry bag. Place the bag in a large drinking glass, flipping the edge of the bag over the sides of the glass so it stands upright. Scoop your frosting into the bag until two-thirds full, then twist the bag shut, removing excess air. Gently press stars (or whatever shape you've chosen) onto the cake in any pattern of your choosing. Refill the pastry bag as needed, and be sure to keep the frosting cool, as the warmth of your hands on the bag will loosen it. This works best with coconut buttercream or chocolate frostings.

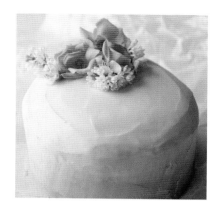

Ombré

This is one of our easier techniques, though we think it looks the most impressive. Simply make some white Coconut Buttercream (page 210), divide it among four small bowls, and follow the instructions on page 210 to create several shades of frosting. Place a pastry bag or resealable plastic bag in a large drinking glass, flipping the edge of the bag over the sides of the glass so it stands up. Scoop the darkest color into the bag, then twist the bag shut, removing excess air. If using a plastic bag, trim off ¼ inch from one corner.

Gently press the frosting around the bottom quarter of the cake, moving the cake platter to help you steady your movement. (Don't worry if it looks a little rough; you'll smooth it out in a minute.) Continue with each color, moving up the cake from darkest to lightest, until you're putting plain white frosting on the top of the cake.

Using your offset spatula, smooth the top of the cake, and then smooth out the sides. You want it to look as flat as possible. Keep rotating the cake platter to get a smooth surface. Use a wet paper towel to wipe any excess frosting off the cake platter.

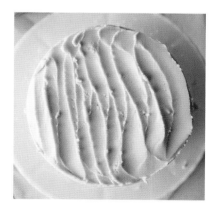

The Swoop

The swoop is the signature Sweet Laurel look, and it's so simple: waves of frosting, accentuating its creamy texture. Frost your cake as cleanly as possible, with at least a ½-inch-thick layer all around. Gently press your offset spatula into the bottom of the side of the cake at a slight angle, about 30 degrees up, just enough to create a wave as you move the spatula. Move the spatula smoothly up; then as it reaches the top lip of the cake, smoothly swoop down. Rotate the cake as you go. Finish by doing the top of the cake, starting the same movement on the far edge of the top, working toward your body. The movement should be rhythmic and fun to do.

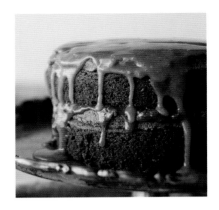

Drizzling

A drizzle can make all the difference between a good-looking cake and an incredible one. If there's a chocolate sauce, caramel, or fruit puree you can work into the cake, drizzle on a bit right before serving, so it clings to the sides as it slides down. We like to do a zigzag pattern across the top of the cake, with nice-sized drips coming off of every angle of the cake.

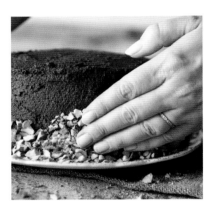

Frosting Coats

Many of our cakes are naked, meaning you can see the layers of cake sandwiching the frosting. But when we want to cover a cake entirely and do something quick and easy for decoration, a coating on the side is just the trick. Choose finely chopped nuts, coconut flakes, or seeds—whatever you think would work well with the cake flavor. Scoop up handfuls and gently press the ingredients into the frosting on the sides of the cake. Continue until the sides of the cake are covered. Simply sweep the excess off of the cake plate before serving.

RESOURCES

Almost all of our ingredients can be found at major retailers (Walmart, Target, Costco, and Whole Foods, for instance), but these are our favorite sources.

Almond Flour: Finding affordable organic almond flour can be a challenge, but Nuts.com is a great source for it, along with conventional almond flour and whole nuts.

Apple Cider Vinegar: Bragg makes a fantastic unfiltered, unheated, and unpasteurized apple cider vinegar.

Arrowroot Powder: Bob's Red Mill's large bag is much more affordable than the small jars you'll find in the spice aisle.

Baking Soda: Bob's Red Mill makes a lovely natural baking soda. It's mined from the ground rather than synthetically created.

Cacao (100% Unsweetened Cacao Powder and 100% Cacao Unsweetened Baking Chocolate): There can be a lot of confusion about what cacao actually is—chocolate is made from cacao. So if you aren't sure, reach for the 100 percent unsweetened chocolate bar and read the label. If the ingredients consist only of cacao, and no sugar, milk, or additives, you're good to go! ChocoVivo's bean-to-bar chocolate factory in Los Angeles is our favorite, but you can find 100 percent bars from more accessible brands like Ghirardelli and Baker's.

Coconut Aminos: This is a delicious gluten- and grain-free substitute for soy sauce made from coconut! It can be found online or at major grocery stores.

Coconut Flour: Bob's Red Mill has a lovely organic version.

Coconut Milk: Finding coconut milk that can whip into thick coconut cream can be a struggle, and a lot of it comes down to picking the right brand. Be sure the coconut milk is in a BPA-free can, is full fat (about 18 percent fat), and contains no additives (these will hurt the milk's ability to whip). We love Natural Value organic coconut milk.

Coconut Oil: For a more delicate flavor and higher cooking temperature, we love Nutiva Refined Coconut Oil. It's steam refined, so no chemicals are used in the process.

Eggs: We always recommend purchasing local, pasture-raised, organic eggs. Our favorite brand is Lily's Eggs, from the Santa Monica Farmer's Market (they are available regionally).

Gelatin: We like Great Lakes Unflavored Beef Gelatin, Collagen Joint Care, the best. It works great and has many nutrients.

Grass-Fed Ghee: 4th and Heart (fourthandheart.com) makes a delicious ghee.

Himalayan Pink Salt: Any brand of pure Himalayan pink salt works for us, as long as it's fine grind.

Honey: We recommend sourcing a local honey from your farmer's market, and raw if noted in recipe.

Maple Syrup: We source our maple syrup from a small Vermont farm, Butternut Mountain Family Farm.

Matcha: Matcha Source (matchasource.com) makes the best matcha latte in town, and their Gotcha Matcha is perfect for our baking needs.

Medjool Dates: The Date Lady (ilovedatelady.com) is a great source for all things dates, including date sugar.

Nut Butter: We make our own nut butters in-house, but love the Once Again brand (onceagainnutbutter.com) when we need to grab a jar for the pantry.

Parchment Paper: We always opt for natural and unbleached parchment paper.

Probiotic Capsules: You can find probiotics in the refrigerator section of health food stores. Be sure to purchase capsules that can be opened, releasing the powder on the inside, and be sure not to use probiotic capsules containing prebiotics, as the fermentation will not occur properly. We like a gluten-free brand called Flora.

Rubber Spatula: For getting into the tight corners of our blender, the silicone ½ spatula by Le Creuset cannot be beat. It's tiny and gets into all of the tight spaces.

Silicone Molds: For cake molds and mats for baking sheets, check out the durable, well-made silicone products from Le Silicone.

Vanilla Bean Powder: Terrasoul makes a great vanilla bean powder; find it online or at health food stores.

Vanilla Extract: If you don't want to make some yourself, try our very own Sweet Laurel grain-free Paleo Vanilla Extract (sweetlaurel.com).

ACKNOWLEDGMENTS

Amanda Englander and the Clarkson Potter team, Laurel and I consider ourselves so fortunate to have you behind us. Thank you for letting us feel like we could take chances and create a cookbook from the heart. You've all been so attentive and collaborative, we couldn't imagine a better team to guide us through creating the first Sweet Laurel cookbook. Alison Fargis, you've been such a fabulous advocate for us from the beginning, and thank you for having our backs every step of the way. You've helped us up our learning curve and encouraged us to create the book we have hoped for since our first phone call, thank you!

From Laurel:

I am grateful for my loving, sweet husband, Nick, and my supportive family, who were my original taste testers and have encouraged me every step of the way throughout life's baking adventures. I'd like to thank my parents for teaching me the value of eating whole foods and how to appreciate the simple beauty found in nature. I would also like to thank Eleanor Womack, MD, who originally diagnosed me, put me on a strict grain-free, refined-sugar-free, and dairy-free diet, and helped me see how attainable healing through food actually is. I'd also like to thank Margaret Floyd (eatnakednow.com), my nutritionist, who continually maneuvers me through the healing process. As a result of her guidance, my autoimmune disease is in remission and I have a healthy and happy baby, Nico. I'd like to thank Sweet Laurel's dedicated customers and fans, who let us know every day that our baked goods have found happy homes (and bellies). And most important, thank you, Claire, for partnering with me in the early stages of Sweet Laurel and sculpting it into the beautiful brand it is today through your creative vision and photography that is unmatched.

From Claire:

I know I'm biased, but I think I have the best family in the world. Mom and Dad, thank you for being so supportive, creative, and encouraging. Amanda, Pat, and Henry, thank you for taste-testing practically every recipe. Aunt Tina, thank you for your help beta testing, and for being my cake inspiration. An especially big thank-you to my husband, Craig, my favorite taste tester and the best partner. You've helped us build Sweet Laurel from an idea to a company with a vision, I couldn't do it without you. I love you. And, even though you were in my belly for most of it, thank you to my son, James, for making the days of recipe testing, shooting, and tasting even more fun.

Kathryn Mauger and Sam Redinger, thank you so much for all of your hard work. You helped make this cookbook the best it could be, and held me up when I was nine months pregnant and still working. Laurel, who could have imagined where that one slice of cake would take us? You are a blessing to me, and not only an amazing partner, a dear friend.

INDEX